Hearing Aid Dispensing
Training Manual

Second Edition

Editor-in-Chief for Audiology
Brad A. Stach, PhD

Hearing Aid Dispensing Training Manual

Second Edition

Suzanne Krumenacker, AuD

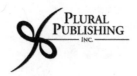

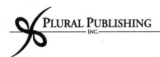
PLURAL PUBLISHING
INC.

5521 Ruffin Road
San Diego, CA 92123

e-mail: information@pluralpublishing.com
Web site: http://www.pluralpublishing.com

Typeset in 10/12 Palatino by Achorn International
Printed in the United States of America by Integrated Books International

Library of Congress Cataloging-in-Publication Data

Names: Krumenacker, Suzanne, author.
Title: Hearing aid dispensing training manual / Suzanne Krumenacker.
Description: Second edition. | San Diego, CA : Plural Publishing, [2019] |
    Includes bibliographical references and index.
Identifiers: LCCN 2018055065 | ISBN 9781635501315 (alk. paper) | ISBN 1635501318
    (alk. paper)
Subjects: | MESH: Hearing Aids | Correction of Hearing Impairment | Professional
    Competence | Hearing Disorders—diagnosis | Deafness—therapy | Hearing Tests
Classification: LCC RF303 | NLM WV 274 | DDC 617.8/9—dc23
LC record available at https://lccn.loc.gov/2018055065

Contents

Preface

The *Hearing Aid Dispensing Training Manual* was developed for those individuals preparing to take their State Hearing Aid Dispensing Practical Examination to obtain their Hearing Aid Dispensing License. This manual is an entry-level, self-paced study guide written for people looking to enter the field of hearing aid dispensing. The purpose of this manual is to complement other material and resources that are currently available to help study for state exams. It is presented in a way so that its main focus is on the areas of competency for the practical sections of the state licensing exams.

The intent of this manual is to assist individuals to not only learn the material for the exam, but also master the material for professional use after passing the examination. The format of this manual is intended to simulate situations presented on most state practical examinations. The manual is laid out in four competency modules, with each module divided into chapters that relate to the concept of the module. Each chapter begins with the objectives and vocabulary, and then proceeds to activities which tie it all together to enable one to perform the tasks proficiently in order to pass the state licensing exam.

WHAT'S NEW TO THE SECOND EDITION

The second edition has revised and updated material thanks to the help and suggestions from previous readers of the first edition. In addition to the first edition updates, there are two new chapters on infection control and tympanometry, module quizzes, cheat sheets, a glossary of terms with definitions, and an abbreviations chart. Another big change comes in Modules 3 and 4, which now include receiver-in-the-canal style devices. You may have also noticed in the bottom right-hand corner of the front cover that there is a box that says "PluralPlus Companion Website." The companion website gives you access to supplemental material that complements the material in the manual. Be sure to look for the companion website icon throughout this manual for more information.

Introduction

The goal for the *Hearing Aid Dispenser Training Manual* is to provide a guide to those individuals who are looking to pursue a career in hearing health care, specifically hearing aid dispensing, who require study material to assist them in preparation for their state's practical (hands-on) licensing examination. This manual is also for those individuals pursuing careers as ototechs, audioprosthologists, audiology assistants, and otolaryngologists who are looking to dispense out of their practice, and those audiologists who need to obtain a hearing aid dispensing license in the state in which they are practicing as a dispensing audiologist.

The purpose of this training manual is to assist candidates in identifying their strengths and weaknesses regarding the content included. This manual is not designed to teach new concepts or information; it assumes that the reader has already studied the information needed for passing the written examination. The goal of this manual is to help put all of the information together in a practical way so that one can proficiently and competently execute the practical sections of the state licensing exam. If you are still in the process of studying the content and have not yet passed your written examination, there is a list of recommended reading material at the end of this manual to help assist you with the core concepts presented here.

There are 18 chapters divided into four modules. Each module represents a core competency that is likely to be presented on any hearing aid dispensing state practical licensing examination. The thought behind this type of module training is that for those states that allow candidates to only retake one section of the practical examination that they did not pass the first time, they will only have to review that one module in this manual. It is, however, highly recommended that you complete the whole manual if you are studying to take the practical examination in your state for the first time.

Since each state regulates its own examinations for licensing, it is also important to note that even if you are licensed in one state and are looking to get licensed in another, you do not automatically have reciprocity in that state and may have to take and pass that state's hearing aid dispensing licensing examination. Review of the four modules in this book will help to direct you to what the states may be looking for that is different from what is done in everyday practice.

Acknowledgments

I thank Candace Myers for being my sounding block, my second set of eyes, and my best friend. I could not have completed this second edition without her and her infinite wisdom. I also thank my family, Ed and Sam, for always supporting me to help me reach my goals. Finally, I thank Plural Publishing for believing in my vision for the second edition of this manual. Thank you for your continued support.

For Candace,
"We will always be friends until we are old and senile. Then, we can be new friends."

MODULE 1

Audiometric Assessment

① Hearing Loss

Objectives

- To prepare the candidate to be familiar with audiometric testing equipment
- To prepare the candidate to be able to recognize different types of audiometric configurations
- To prepare the candidate to be able to identify the three main characteristics of a hearing loss
- To prepare the candidate to be able to discuss different characteristics of an audiogram

TERMS AND DEFINITIONS

Air conduction: the process by which sound travels to the inner ear and brain by way of the outer ear to the middle ear

Air–bone gap: a name given to denote the difference in hearing sensitivity between bone conduction and air conduction thresholds

Bone conduction: the process by which sound travels to the inner ear and brain by way of the mastoid process, bypassing the outer and middle ear

Hearing loss: refers to the partial or total inability to hear sounds in one or both ears

Retrocochlear: everything after the cochlea, that is, auditory nerve and brain

Please refer to the glossary in the back of this book for more terms and definitions.

THE AUDIOMETER

Audiometry is a procedure that measures a person's hearing sensitivity by way of an audiometer, relative to the sensitivity of average hearing. An audiometer is an instrument used for measuring hearing thresholds using both air and bone conduction methods. All audiometers have two main controls that are fairly standard, the frequency control and an intensity control. Most frequency controls allow you to test 125, 250, 500, 750, 1000, 1500, 2000, 3000, 4000, 6000, and 8000 Hz. There are some audiometers that can test ultrahigh frequencies up to 20,000 Hz, but for standard pure-tone testing on state examinations, the range of 250 to 8000 Hz is sufficient unless your state says otherwise. The intensity control on the audiometer generally allows you to test between −10 dB HL and 110 dB HL; however, there are some audiometers that have extended ranges and can test even higher. Figure 1–1, Figure 1–2, and Figure 1–3 provide examples of a portable audiometer, headphones, and a bone oscillator, respectively.

All audiometers are different and can vary from manufacturer to manufacturer, and because of this, they can function very differently. You may see stimulus controls which allow you to choose between pure tone, warble, and speech stimulus. You may

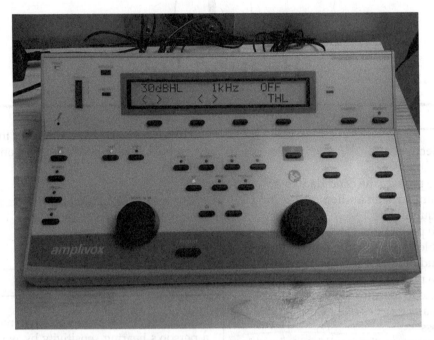

Figure 1–1. An example of a two-channel portable audiometer is shown. (Courtesy of Suzanne Krumenacker)

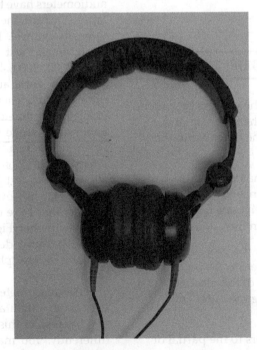

Figure 1–2. An example of a set of headphones is shown. (Courtesy of Suzanne Krumenacker)

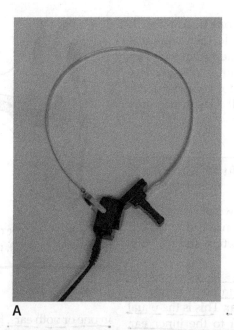

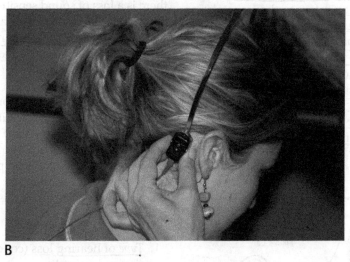

Figure 1–3. A. A bone conduction oscillator and headband are shown. (Courtesy of Suzanne Krumenacker) **B.** Bone conduction oscillator placement on a patient. (From Valente, 2009, p. 28)

also have a separate control for masking noise that can be presented using a continuous or pulsating tone. Be familiar with standard controls, and if you have an audiometer that you can practice on, take the time to know the function of each button and switch. It is always best and recommended to consult the user manual for a particular audiometer on the specific functions of that instrument.

For state licensing examinations, individual states may require you to bring your own audiometer to the practical exam. If that is the case in your state, then you must read the requirements of the audiometer that the state provides to ensure that a particular audiometer will work for your exam. For example, some states will let you use only two-channel audiometers.

DESCRIBING THE AUDIOGRAM

In normal ears there are two possible routes for sound to travel, as shown in Figure 1–4 and Figure 1–5: (1) air conduction and (2) bone conduction.

Air conduction refers to the transmission of sound waves from air through the middle ear to the inner ear. This is the usual route of sound to travel to the inner ear. Bone conduction refers to the transmission of acoustic signals through the mastoid or frontal bone of the skull. The signal is directed into the inner ear only, bypassing the outer and middle parts of the ear.

Normal hearing occurs when sound is conducted efficiently through the outer, middle, and inner ear, and hearing loss refers to the partial or total inability to hear sounds

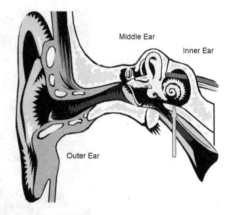

Figure 1–5. The bone conduction pathway is shown. (From Valente, 2009, p. 29)

in one or both ears. Hearing loss occurs when there is a loss of sound sensitivity because of an abnormality somewhere along the auditory pathway. An example of normal hearing is when *all* air and bone conduction thresholds are better than 25 dB HL (discussed later in this chapter).

By performing an audiometric test, we are able to determine the different characteristics of a hearing loss if one presents. When a hearing test is performed, there are general characteristics that present, which are used when discussing or describing the hearing loss. A hearing loss is characterized by three descriptors:

1. *Type* of hearing loss (conductive, sensorineural, mixed)
2. *Degree* of hearing loss (mild, moderate, severe, profound)
3. *Configuration* of the hearing loss, what the hearing loss looks like (e.g., flat, sloping, cookie-bite, rising or reverse slope, corner audiogram, ski-slope, noise-notch)

Types of Hearing Loss

The first characteristic that we discuss is *type* of hearing loss. When discussing the type of

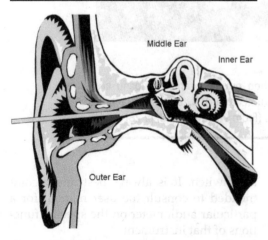

Figure 1–4. The air conduction pathway is shown. (From Valente, 2009, p. 26)

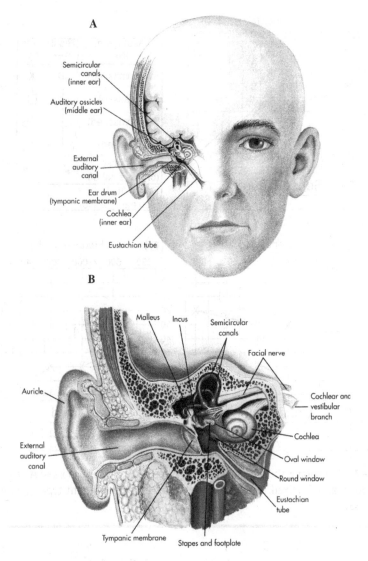

A

Semicircular
canals
(inner ear)

Auditory ossicles
(middle ear)

External
auditory
canal

Ear drum
(tympanic membrane)

Cochlea
(inner ear)

Eustachian tube

B

Malleus   Incus

Semicircular
canals

Facial nerve

Auricle

Cochlear and
vestibular
branch

External
auditory
canal

Cochlea

Oval window

Round window

Eustachian
tube

Tympanic membrane   Stapes and footplate

Figure 1–6. A. Orientation of auditory and vestibular structures in the human skull. **B.** Coronal view of the auditory and vestibular structures. (From Seidal, Ball, Dains, & Benedict, 2003)

hearing loss, we speak in terms of whether it is considered *conductive, sensorineural,* or *mixed*. A *conductive* hearing loss is a loss that occurs when sound is not transmitted efficiently through the ear canal, eardrum, and ossicles of the middle ear. In short, *a conductive loss is a hearing loss occurring anywhere in the outer or middle ear.* See Figure 1–6 for general anatomy of the ear for reference.

A *conductive hearing loss* may be caused by conditions such as middle or outer ear infection, perforated tympanic membrane, impacted cerumen, benign tumors, or absence or malformation of the outer ear, ear canal, or middle ear. This type of hearing loss *can* often be medically or surgically treated. Bone conduction thresholds are significantly better than air conduction thresholds and within normal

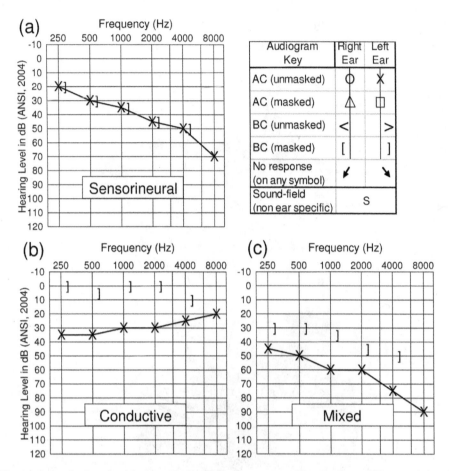

Figure 1–7. Audiograms show examples of the three types of hearing losses: A. sensorineural, B. conductive, and C. mixed. See text for definitions of the different types. (From Kramer, 2008, p. 153)

range on the audiogram when a *conductive* hearing loss is present. That is known as an air–bone gap. See Figure 1–7 for an example of a conductive hearing loss on an audiogram.

Air–Bone Gap

- An air–bone gap always presents with better hearing by bone conduction than air conduction.
- An air–bone gap indicates a blockage or impairment to the conductive portion of the hearing mechanism (outer or middle ears).

- If there is an air–bone gap of 15 dB or more at all frequencies, you have a conductive hearing loss or a conductive component.

The next type of hearing loss that we discuss is a *sensorineural hearing loss.* A sensorineural hearing loss occurs when there is damage to the inner ear (cochlea) or to the nerve pathways from the inner ear to the brain (retrocochlear). A sensorineural hearing loss can be caused by disease, birth injury, drugs that are toxic to the auditory system, genetic syndromes, noise exposure, viruses, head trauma, aging, and tumors. This type of hearing loss cannot be medically or surgically corrected, and is a permanent loss. On an audiogram, the configuration of a sensorineural hearing loss is when the air conduction thresholds and bone conduction thresholds are the same (right on top of each other on the audiogram), as shown in Figure 1–7.

The third and final type of hearing loss to discuss is a *mixed hearing loss*. Sometimes a conductive hearing loss occurs in combination with a sensorineural hearing loss. This type of hearing loss is referred to as a mixed hearing loss when there is damage to the outer or middle ears *and* the inner ear (cochlea) or auditory nerve. With a mixed hearing loss there is a separation between the air conduction thresholds and bone conduction thresholds in addition to abnormal bone conduction thresholds (worse than 20 dB on the audiogram), as seen in Figure 1–7.

Degrees of Hearing Loss

The second characteristic of hearing loss that we discuss is *degree* of hearing loss. Degree of hearing loss refers to the severity of the loss. There are six broad categories that are typically used. The numbers are representative of the patient's thresholds, or the softest sound that the patient can perceive. One accepted scale that is used for description of the degree of hearing loss and how it affects communication is given below (Clark, 1981):

Normal	−10 to 15 dB HL
Normal for adults; slight for children	16 to 25 dB HL
Mild	26 to 40 dB HL
Moderate	41 to 55 dB HL
Moderately severe	56 to 70 dB HL
Severe	71 to 90 dB HL
Profound	91+ dB HL

Configurations of Hearing Loss

The third and final characteristic of hearing loss is the *configuration* of the hearing loss. The configuration or shape of the hearing loss refers to: (1) the extent of hearing loss at each frequency and (2) the overall picture of hearing that is created. For example, a hearing loss that only affects the high frequencies would be described as a *ski-slope loss* or a *high-frequency loss*. Its configuration would show good hearing in the low frequencies and poor hearing in the high frequencies. The following descriptions and illustrations are examples of the most common configurations of hearing loss and what they look like on an audiogram:

- Flat loss: Generally varies within 10 to 15 dB at all frequencies
- Gently sloping: A gradual reduction from lower to higher frequencies
- Rising or reverse slope: Greater hearing loss in the low frequencies, better hearing in the highs
- Corner audiogram: Severe to profound loss in the low frequencies, no response in the mid or high frequencies
- Ski-slope, high-frequency, or precipitous loss: Better hearing in low-frequency range to a severe drop in the highs
- Noise-notch: A common audiogram configuration for people with hearing loss due to noise exposure. Commonly seen with this loss is what is known as a noise-induced notch, which is a sensorineural hearing loss with maximum loss typically between 3000 and 6000 Hz, as shown in Figure 1–8.

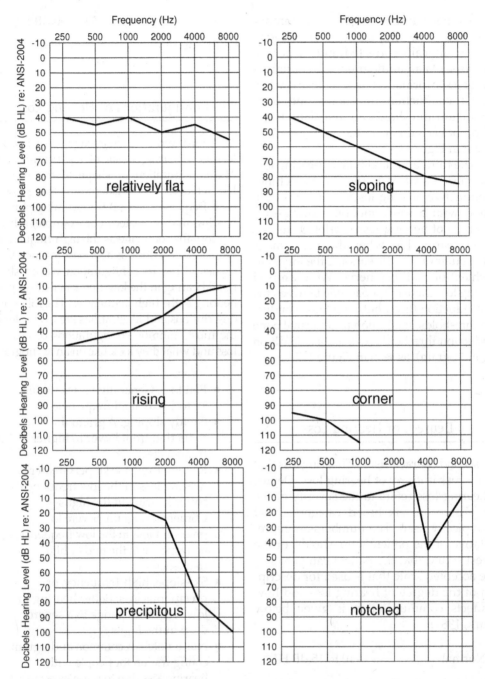

Figure 1–8. Audiogram configurations with common terms used to describe their shapes. See text for definitions of the terms. (From Kramer, 2008, p. 154)

Other terms and descriptors with which to be familiar, and which are discussed more in Chapter 2, are as follows:

Unilateral hearing loss	Loss of hearing in only one ear
Bilateral hearing loss	Loss of hearing in both ears
Fluctuating hearing loss	Hearing loss that is always changing over time
Stable hearing loss	No change in hearing over time
Sudden hearing loss	Loss of hearing that occurs quickly
Progressive hearing loss	Loss of hearing that presents slowly over time
Symmetrical hearing loss	The characteristics of degree and configuration of the loss are the same in both ears
Asymmetrical hearing loss	The characteristics of degree and configuration of the loss are different between ears

REFERENCES

Clark, J. G. (1981). Uses and abuses of hearing loss classification. *ASHA, 23*, 493–500.

Kramer, S. (2008). *Audiology: Science to practice.* San Diego, CA: Plural Publishing.

Seidal, H. M., Ball, J. W., Dains, J. E., & Benedict, G. W. (2003). *Mosby's guide to physical examination* (p. 314). Amsterdam, Netherlands: Elsevier.

Valente, M. (2009). *Pure-tone audiometry and masking.* San Diego, CA: Plural Publishing.

Audiogram Interpretation

TERMS AND DEFINITIONS

Audiogram: a standard graph that shows hearing-threshold levels as a function of frequency

Conductive hearing loss: a loss that occurs when sound is not transmitted efficiently through the outer and middle ear

Mixed hearing loss: a hearing loss that has both conductive and sensorineural components

Sensorineural hearing loss: hearing loss caused when there is damage to the inner ear (cochlea) or to the nerve pathways from the inner ear to the brain

Threshold: the softest level that someone can hear 50% of the time

Please refer to the glossary at the end of this book for more terms and definitions.

UNDERSTANDING THE AUDIOGRAM

In Chapter 1 we focused on the different characteristics of hearing loss. In this chapter we focus on the audiogram itself. When "interpreting an audiogram," we are looking at the audiogram and describing the hearing loss. As discussed in the previous chapter, we look at three things:

1. Type of hearing loss (conductive, sensorineural, mixed)
2. Degree of hearing loss (mild, moderate, severe, profound)
3. Configuration (flat, sloping, corner, etc.)

When determining the type, degree, and configuration of a hearing loss, we need to be able to read and interpret the audiogram in order to describe and understand what we are seeing.

The Audiogram

An audiogram is an audiometric worksheet in which the patient's hearing thresholds are recorded for each frequency. Figure 2–1 is what a typical audiogram looks like with the frequencies listed on the top and the hearing level in decibel hearing level (dB HL) listed along the left side. The audiogram typically consists of other important information recorded on it, such as patient name, age, sex, date of the exam, equipment used (audiometer/earphone type), test reliability, and comments, as well as the hearing test information. In some states, you may be required to sign the audiogram and provide your hearing aid dispensing license number as well. Every audiogram has a key for the symbols used for marking your results. Typically, clinicians use a red pen (for the right ear) and a blue pen (for the left ear) when recording the symbols. Using different color

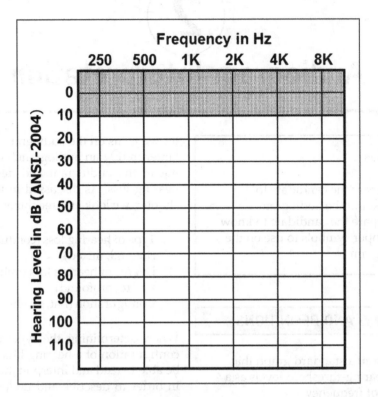

Figure 2–1. A typical audiogram is shown. (From DeRuiter & Ramachandran, 2010)

pens is helpful during counseling the patient because it makes it easier for the patient to distinguish between the ears when you are explaining to her/him the audiometric test results. If red and blue pens are provided by your state during your exam, make sure you use them when marking your audiogram to denote the proper ears.

Most symbols are universal, but there are some that can vary (Figure 2–2). When taking your state exam, read the information that the state provides for the audiometric assessment and be sure to note if the state recommends using particular symbols.

Examples of how symbols can vary are often seen when marking a patient's Uncomfortable Loudness Level (UCL) or Threshold of Discomfort (TD). If you are testing using pure tones, you need to mark the level on the audiogram on the particular frequency tested just as you would your air conduc-

tion and bone conduction scores. If you are told to mark the threshold a certain way by your state, then follow its instructions. Some varying symbols that are used for Threshold of Discomfort are TD, U, UCL, LDL (loudness discomfort level), and so forth. If testing using speech, you would mark the dB HL that is obtained for each ear in the box provided on the audiogram. If no instruction is given, then use the symbol provided on your audiogram.

So what does the hearing loss look like on paper? Figure 2–3, Figure 2–4, and Figure 2–5 illustrate what the following types of hearing losses "look like" on an audiogram:

Sensorineural hearing loss—symbols representing thresholds for air and bone conduction are on top of each other on the audiogram.

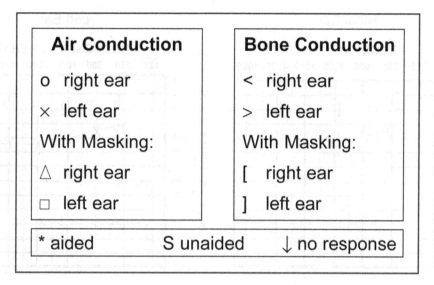

Figure 2–2. Figure legend for an audiogram is shown. (From DeRuiter & Ramachandran, 2010)

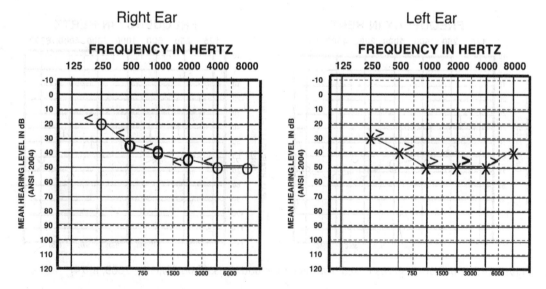

Figure 2–3. Audiogram shows sensorineural hearing loss in both ears. (From Valente, 2009, p. 75)

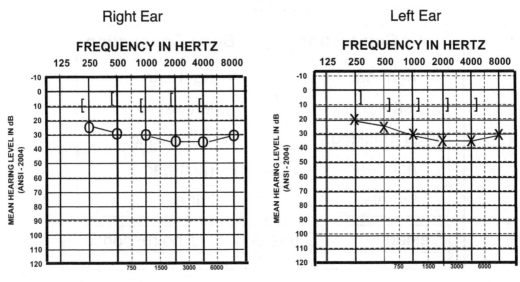

Figure 2–4. Audiogram shows conductive hearing loss in both ears. (From Valente, 2009, p. 74)

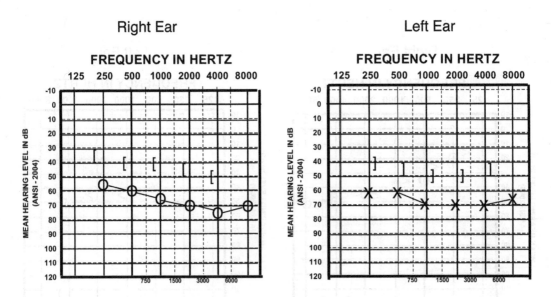

Figure 2–5. Audiogram shows mixed hearing loss in both ears. (From Valente, 2009, p. 74)

Conductive hearing loss—symbols representing thresholds for air conduction are 25 dB HL or poorer, and the bone conduction thresholds are normal.

Mixed hearing loss—symbols representing both air and bone conduction are impaired, and bone conduction thresholds are significantly better than air conduction by 15 db HL or more.

Other descriptors associated with hearing loss are:

Bilateral versus unilateral. Bilateral hearing loss means both ears are affected. Unilateral hearing loss means only one ear is affected.

Symmetrical versus asymmetrical. Symmetrical hearing loss means that the degree and configuration of hearing loss are the same in each ear. An asymmetrical hearing loss is one in which the degree and/or configuration of the loss is different for each ear.

Progressive versus sudden hearing loss. Progressive hearing loss becomes increasingly worse over time. A sudden hearing loss is one that has an acute or rapid onset and therefore occurs quickly, requiring immediate medical attention to determine its cause and treatment.

Fluctuating versus stable hearing loss. Some hearing losses change—sometimes getting better, sometimes getting worse. Fluctuating hearing loss is typically a symptom of conductive hearing loss caused by ear infection and middle ear fluid, but also presents in other conditions, such as Ménière's disease.

EXAMPLES OF AUDIOGRAM AND DESCRIPTIONS

The examples in Figure 2–6, Figure 2–7, Figure 2–8, Figure 2–9, and Figure 2–10 are provided to ensure that you are familiar with being able to read and describe audiogram

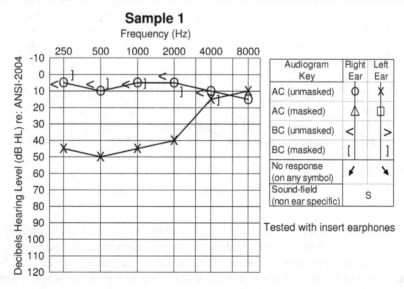

Figure 2–6. Audiogram sample 1. Two possible descriptions of the audiogram are: (a) pure-tone loss through 2000 Hz rising to normal in the higher frequencies for the left ear. Hearing was within normal limits for the right ear. (b) The left ear showed a moderate conductive hearing loss through 2000 Hz. (From Kramer, 2008, p. 155)

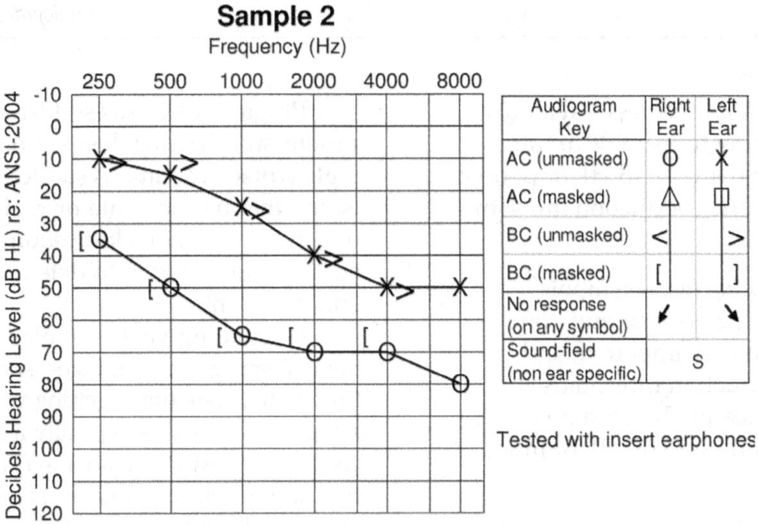

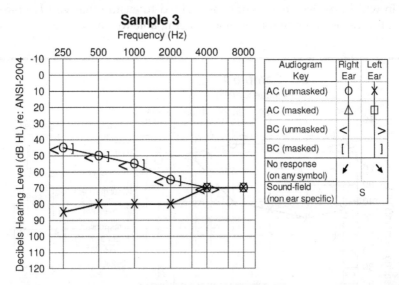

Figure 2–7. Audiogram sample 2. Two possible descriptions of the audiogram are: (a) pure-tone threshold testing for the left ear indicated a sensorineural hearing loss that was mild at 1000 Hz sloping to moderate in the higher frequencies. The right ear showed a sloping sensorineural hearing loss that was mild at 250 Hz sloping to severe at 8000 Hz. (b) The left ear has mild to moderate high-frequency sensorineural hearing loss with normal hearing in the lower frequencies. The right ear has a mild to moderate sensorineural hearing loss through 500 Hz sloping to severe at 8000 Hz. (From Kramer, 2008, p. 156)

Figure 2–8. Audiogram sample 3. Two possible descriptions of the audiogram are: (a) pure-tone threshold testing indicated a moderate to moderately severe sloping sensorineural hearing loss in the right ear. The left ear showed a severe, relatively flat, mixed hearing loss through 2000 Hz (with 40 dB air–bone gap at 250 to 15 dB air–bone gap at 2000 Hz), rising to a moderately severe sensorineural hearing loss in the higher frequencies. (b) The right ear has a sloping sensorineural hearing loss that ranges from moderate in the low frequencies to moderately severe in the mid to high frequencies. The left ear has a severe, flat hearing loss with a conductive (air–bone gap) component from 250 to 2000 Hz. (From Kramer, 2008, p. 157)

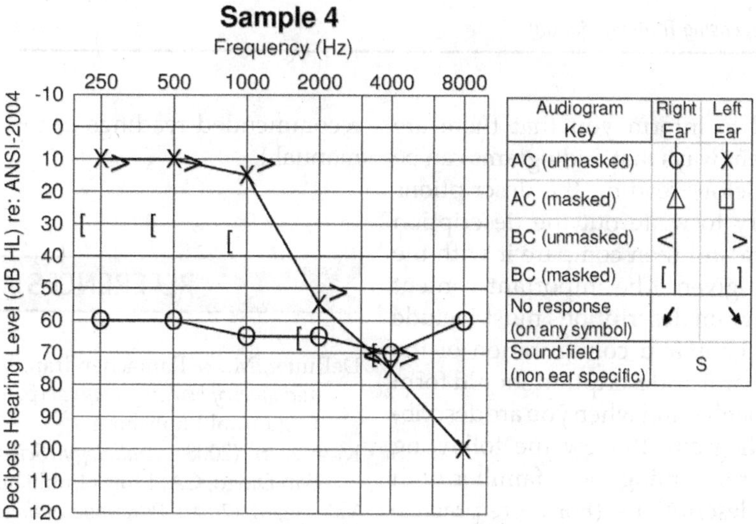

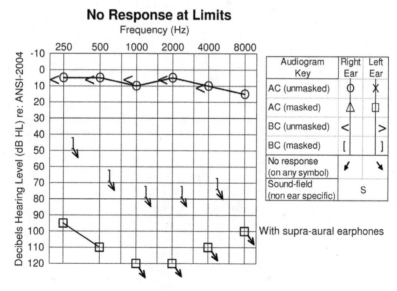

Sample 4

Figure 2–9. Audiogram sample 4. Two possible descriptions of the audiogram are: (a) pure-tone threshold testing indicated a relatively flat, moderately severe hearing loss in the right ear, which was mixed (30 dB air–bone gaps) through 1000 Hz and sensorineural from 2000 to 8000 Hz. The left ear has normal hearing through 1000 Hz with a sensorineural hearing loss that precipitously slopes to severe at 4000 Hz and profound at 8000 Hz. (b) the right ear has a moderately severe mixed hearing loss through 1000 Hz (30 dB air–bone gaps) and a moderately severe sensorineural hearing loss in the higher frequencies. The left ear has a moderate to profound sloping sensorineural hearing loss from 2000 to 8000 Hz. (From Kramer, 2008, p. 158)

Figure 2–10. An example of an audiogram shows no responses at the limits of the equipment for the left ear bone conduction and air conduction thresholds. The appropriate symbols have an arrow attached to indicate that testing was performed up to the indicated maximum limit, but the patient did not respond at those levels. The difference between the air conduction and bone conduction symbols does not imply any air–bone gaps, since the actual thresholds for the left ear are not able to be determined due to output limits of the transducers. The patient has a hearing loss in the left ear that is greater than was able to be tested. This audiogram might be described as having no usable hearing in the left ear. (From Kramer, 2008, p. 159)

results, and to inform you that there are many different ways that audiograms can be described. Before reading the descriptions provided, try to write out the description on your own and then compare it with the descriptions given. The important content in the audiogram descriptions must include the type, degree, and configuration of the loss in each ear. The description should form a picture in one's mind when you are describing the audiogram. Review the following examples for becoming more familiar with audiogram descriptions. (For more practice on audiogram interpretation, refer to the recommended readings in the back of this manual.)

REFERENCES

DeRuiter, M., & Ramachandran, V. (2010). *Basic audiometry learning manual* (p. 86). San Diego, CA: Plural Publishing.

Kramer, S. (2008). *Audiology: Science to practice*. San Diego, CA: Plural Publishing.

Valente, M. (2009). *Pure-tone audiometry and masking*. San Diego, CA: Plural Publishing.

3

FDA Red Flags

Objectives

- To prepare the candidate to be able to recognize disorders of the ear
- To prepare the candidate to know when to refer or not refer the patient for medical evaluation
- To prepare the candidate to know the eight FDA red flags

TERMS AND DEFINITIONS

Anotia: complete absence of the auricle

Atresia: complete closure of the external auditory canal

Congenital: to be born with something

FDA: Food and Drug Administration

Microtia: a very tiny external auditory canal that is congenital in nature

Otalgia: pain in the ear

Otorrhea: any discharge from the outer or middle ear

Stenosis: narrowing of the external auditory canal

Please refer to the glossary at the end of this book for more terms and definitions.

TO REFER OR NOT TO REFER, THAT IS THE QUESTION!

It is our professional responsibility to know when to refer, or not to refer, a patient, and we need to think about pathology within our scope of practice when it comes to hearing aid dispensing. The provisions that are discussed in this chapter are safeguards to the consumers so that they know that any and all medical treatments will be attempted first before hearing aids are recommended. The following is the Food and Drug Administration's (FDA) hearing aid fitting referral criteria, established in 1977, also known as the FDA's eight "red flags," which you should commit to memory, as this is almost guaranteed to be part of your state licensing exam.

The FDA's Eight Red Flags

1. Visible congenital or traumatic deformity of the ear
2. History of active drainage from the ear in the previous 90 days
3. History of sudden or rapidly progressive hearing loss within the previous 90 days
4. Acute or chronic dizziness
5. Unilateral hearing loss of sudden or recent onset within the previous 90 days
6. Audiometric air–bone gap equal to or greater than 15 dB at 500, 1000, and 2000 Hz
7. Visible evidence of significant cerumen accumulation or a foreign body in the ear canal
8. Pain or discomfort in the ear

Cheat sheet provided in Appendix F.

PATHOLOGIES RELATED TO THE FDA'S EIGHT RED FLAGS

Disorders of the Outer, Middle, and Inner Ear

Once you become a licensed hearing aid dispenser, you cannot state the cause of a hearing loss, nor can you diagnose the hearing loss, but you can and must be able to know and recognize the different types of hearing loss as discussed in Chapters 1 and 2. When someone walks into your office for a hearing test, he or she may be experiencing several symptoms. What are the possible symptoms? Hearing loss, tinnitus, dizziness, fullness, sensitivity to sound, pain, drainage, discomfort, trouble hearing in noise, itchy ears, inflammation, and so forth. It is important to know to what the symptoms that they are reporting could be attributed. Most common hearing disorders can be broken down into three major parts: outer, middle, and inner ear, and in turn they correlate in some way to the FDA's red flags. Table 3–1 provides a breakdown of the different disorders with a disorder description, type of hearing loss, treatment options, and tympanogram type. This table will also provide useful information for upcoming chapters in this module.

Primary Disorders of the Outer Ear

Malformations of the Auricle/Pinna and External Auditory Canal. Although malformations of the auricle and external auditory canal can occur for many reasons, the most common are congenital malformations such as microtia, atresia, and stenosis. Accidents or surgery where a portion of the auricle has been removed, or the auricle is missing completely, is known as anotia. Although malformations of the auricle do not generally cause a hearing loss, those affecting the external auditory canal can. Figure 3–1 shows the different landmarks of a healthy ear.

Impacted Cerumen. Impacted cerumen is earwax in the canal, which can cause a hearing loss if the amount of wax is substantial enough to block the sound from traveling to the middle and inner ear.

Eczema or Dermatitis. Eczema or dermatitis causes inflammation of the skin in the external auditory canal, which can become red, itchy, and swollen.

External Otitis. External otitis is an infection that forms in the skin of the external auditory canal that is frequently seen in swimmers and people who have water trapped in the ear canal.

Other Disorders of the Outer Ear

In order to discuss the following disorders, we first need to understand and be familiar with what a normal healthy tympanic membrane (TM) looks like along with the landmarks that can be visualized. Figure 3–2 shows a healthy, normal TM. You will notice that the "cone of light" is visible in the lower inferior anterior quadrant at about 5 o'clock. You can often use the cone of light as an important landmark to orient yourself when performing an otoscopic examination (DeRuiter & Ramachandran, 2010, p. 14). Other landmarks that are seen in a healthy, normal ear canal are presented in Figure 3–3.

Polyps. Polyps are growths in the external auditory canal (Figure 3–4).

Perforation of the Tympanic Membrane. Perforations of the TM can occur for many different reasons. They can be caused by infection in the middle ear where pressure builds up, causing the TM to rupture. Direct trauma to the TM can cause perforations and punctures by things such as cotton swabs or paper clips, as well as loud explosions near the ear or a pressure change in

Table 3–1. Disorders of the Ear (Courtesy of Suzanne Krumenacker)

Type of Hearing Loss	Treatment	Description	Tympanogram	ETC
N/A	Surgery	Complete absence of the auricle	A	
Conductive	Surgery	Complete closure of the EAC	Cannot test	
Conductive	Surgery	Very small size of ear	A	
Conductive	Observation/surgery	Narrowing of the canal	A	
Conductive	Removal	Varied amount	A or B	Cannot test if impacted
Conductive	Medical treatment	Infection of the skin in the EAC	A or B	
Conductive	Removal	Objects that fit in the EAC that don't belong	A or B	Cannot test if ear canal is completely blocked
Conductive	Observation/surgery	Bony growths in the EAC	A or B	Depending on the size of the growth
Conductive	Observation/surgery	Hole in the TM due to OM, trauma, infection	B	
Conductive	Hearing aids/surgery	Thickening of the TM by calcium buildup	As	
Conductive	Hearing aids/surgery	Ossicles become altered and do not function properly together	Ad	
Conductive	Medical treatment	Inflammation of the middle ear	B or C	B (with fluid) or C (no fluid, negative pressure)
Conductive	Medical treatment	Inflammation of the middle ear with fluid	B	
Conductive/mixed (Carhart's notch)	Hearing aids/surgery	Bony growth that occurs around the stapes footplate causing it to not move	As	
Conductive	Hearing aids/surgery	Ossicles become ossified and unable to move	As	
Conductive	Surgery	Growth in the middle ear and/or mastoid		

Table 3–1. *Continued*

Type of Hearing Loss	Treatment	Description	Tympanogram	ETC
Sensorineural	Hearing aids	Exposure to a sudden loud sound traumatizing the inner ear	A	
Sensorineural (possible fluctuations)	Medical treatment/ hearing aids	A disease of the inner ear that is caused by an excess of endolymph fluid	A	
Sensorineural	Hearing aids	Progressive hearing loss due to history of noise exposure	A	
Sensorineural	Hearing aids	Hearing loss that is caused by drugs that are toxic to the ear	A	
Sensorineural	Surgery/hearing aids	Slow growing benign tumor or unknown cause	A	Generally unilateral

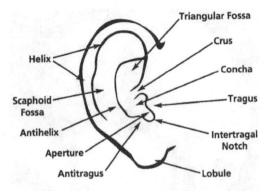

Figure 3–1. The landmarks of the pinna are shown. (From Taylor & Mueller, 2011)

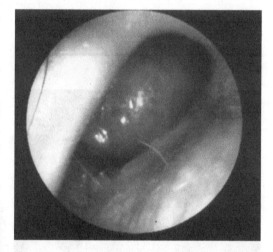

Figure 3–3. Drawing of a tympanic membrane. (From Pasha, 2011)

the external ear canal. An example of a perforated TM is given in Figure 3–5.

Foreign Objects in the Ear Canal. At times a foreign object can get into the ear canal. Such a foreign object could be, for example, an insect, cotton, an eraser, and so forth. If any of these objects make their way into the bony portion of the ear canal, this may result

Figure 3–4. Large polyp occupying the medial portion of the external auditory canal secondary to a cholesteatoma. (From Touma & Touma, 2006, p. 80)

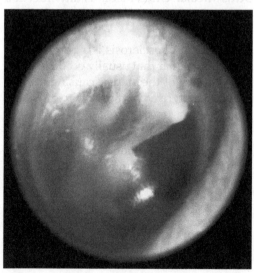

Figure 3–2. Normal tympanic membrane. The umbo is seen in the middle of the tympanic membrane and the "cone of light" is visualized at about 5 o'clock. (From Touma & Touma, 2006, p. 7)

in some swelling of the canal wall and the object will need to be medically removed. See Figure 3–6 and Figure 3–7 for examples of foreign bodies that can accidentally enter the external ear canal.

Exostoses. An example of exostoses is given in Figure 3–8. Exostoses are bony growths that occur in the ear canal and can vary in size and location. These bony growths more times than not are harmless, but at times

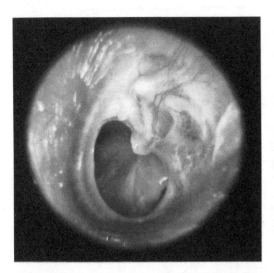

Figure 3–5. Perforation of the tympanic membrane is shown. (From Touma & Touma, 2006, p. 129)

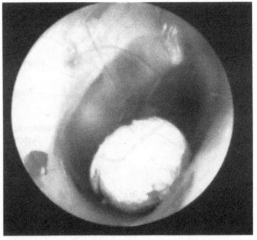

Figure 3–7. A foreign body, a pearl, is shown. (From Touma & Touma, 2006, p. 174)

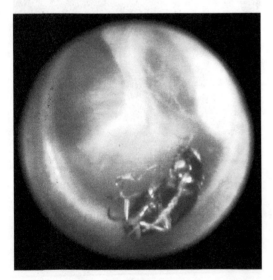

Figure 3–6. A foreign body, a bug, is shown. (From Touma & Touma, 2006, p. 168)

they can cause trouble when performing an audiometric test, and they also have the potential for causing issues during impression taking and the fitting of a hearing aid (DeRuiter & Ramachandran, 2010, p. 16).

Disorders of the Middle Ear

Tympanosclerosis. Generally occurring secondary to a middle ear infection, calcium can build up on the TM, causing it to become thickened, a condition known as tympanosclerosis.

Otitis Media. Otitis media is any infection occurring in the middle ear (Figure 3–9).

Otosclerosis. Otosclerosis is a bony growth in the middle ear that usually occurs around the footplate of the stapes, causing the stapes to remain fixed and unable to move.

Ossicular Discontinuity. Ossicular discontinuity is where the bones of the middle ear become altered, causing them to not function properly together.

Ossicular Fixation. Ossicular fixation is when the bones of the middle ear become ossified and unable to move.

Cholesteatoma. Cholesteatoma is a tumor that occurs in the middle ear and/or mastoid (Figure 3–10).

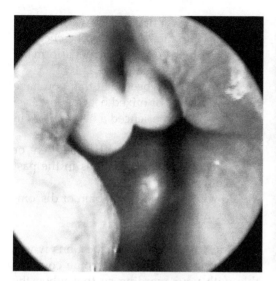

Figure 3–8. Exostosis of the ear canal is shown. (From Touma & Touma, 2006, p. 148)

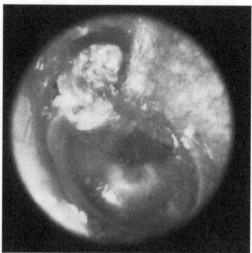

Figure 3–10. Attic-retraction cholesteatoma with extension along the posterior surface of the handle of the malleus medial to the tympanic cavity. (From Touma & Touma, 2006, p. 109)

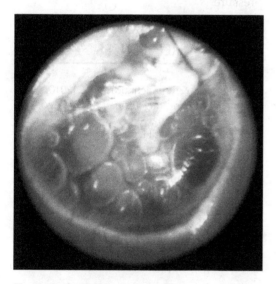

Figure 3–9. Bubbles in the middle ear are shown. (From Touma & Touma, 2006, p. 12)

Disorders of the Inner Ear

Acoustic Trauma. Acoustic trauma is sudden exposure to a loud sound traumatizing the inner ear and causing permanent damage.

Noise-Induced Hearing Loss. Noise-induced hearing loss is exposure to loud sounds over a long period of time, causing permanent damage to the inner ear.

Tinnitus. Tinnitus is noise in the ear that has been described as buzzing, ringing, chirping, and hissing.

Ménière's Disease. Ménière's disease is a disease of the inner ear that is caused by an excess of endolymph fluid and is often accompanied by symptoms such as fluctuating hearing loss, dizziness, and tinnitus.

Acoustic Neuroma. Acoustic neuroma is a tumor that develops in the auditory nerve.

Ototoxicity. Ototoxicity is a hearing loss that occurs by taking drugs that are poisonous to the ear.

REMEMBERING THE RED FLAGS

Here is a trick that I have used over the years with people I have trained to help them remember the FDA's eight red flags, so that when you get into the Practical Exam and the nerves start kicking in, it can be an easy way for you to remember the red flags. I call it "Triple D, Double C, UPS," and it goes like this:

- D—Drainage
- D—Deformity
- D—Dizziness
- C—Cerumen
- C—Conductive component
- U—Unilateral hearing loss
- P—Pain
- S—Sudden hearing loss

Most states require you to ask the questions during our exam to ensure that you are aware of the reasons you would need to refer for medical evaluation. Below are examples of how you can ask the questions in relation to the "Triple D, Double C, UPS":

1. I will be looking at your ears for any visible signs of abnormality when I perform the otoscopic examination. Have you had any surgery or trauma to your ears in the past?
2. Have you experienced drainage from your ears in the past 90 days?
3. Have you been experiencing any dizziness?
4. Have you ever had to have wax removed from your ears? I will also be checking for cerumen buildup when I perform the otoscopic examination.
5. Have you ever been told that you have a conductive or mixed hearing loss?
6. Have you experienced a hearing loss in only one ear?
7. Have you experienced a sudden or rapid onset of hearing loss in the past 90 days?
8. Do you experience any pain or discomfort in your ears?

Practice asking these questions whenever you have a chance. Become comfortable with your wording so that when the time comes that you have to ask the questions during your examination, it will be second nature and you will not forget under pressure.

REFERENCES

DeRuiter, M., & Ramachandran, V. (2010). *Basic audiometry learning manual*. San Diego, CA: Plural Publishing.

Taylor, B., & Mueller, H. G. (2011). *Fitting and dispensing hearing aids* (p. 48). San Diego, CA: Plural Publishing.

Touma, J., & Touma, B. (2006). *Atlas of otoscopy*. San Diego, CA: Plural Publishing.

US Food and Drug Administration. (1977, February 15). Rules and regulations regarding hearing aid devices: Professional and patient labeling and conditions for sale, Part IV. *Federal Registers*, pp. 9286–9296.

Infection Control

TERMS AND DEFINITIONS

Cleaning: the process of removing debris, decreasing the number of microorganisms that are present

Cross-contamination: the passing of bacteria, microorganisms, or other harmful substances indirectly from one patient to another through improper or unsterile procedures, equipment, hearing aids, or earmolds

Disinfecting: the process of killing most germs by using a disinfectant by either spraying it on the surface or immersing it

Standard precautions: a set of infection control practices used to prevent transmission of diseases that can be acquired by contact with blood, body fluids, non-intact skin (including rashes), and mucous membranes

Infectious disease: caused by the entrance into the body of organisms (as bacteria, protozoans, fungi, or viruses) which grow and multiply there

Sterilizing: the process of removing 100% of the microorganisms and their spores so that they cannot reproduce

Please refer to the glossary at the end of this book for more terms and definitions.

OVERVIEW

Just as it is our professional responsibility to know when to refer a patient as we discussed in the previous chapter, it is also our professional responsibility to ensure our patients' safety as well as our own when it comes to preventing the spread of infectious disease. This chapter is meant to be an introduction to the effective methods and best practices of infection control. For your state exam, patients' safety is taken very serious and is generally the #1 priority. With that being said, it is your responsibility to know which areas of your practice can affect your patient (as well as yourself), because those areas will be looked at as a high priority on your state exam. Because the methods and practices of infection control are always changing, it can be difficult to stay updated. At the end of this chapter, you will find multiple references, resources, and website links to those institutions that set forth the requirements for infection control. Most importantly, check your state website for more information and what may be pertinent to you for your state licensing exam.

Before we begin this chapter, ask yourself this question and please answer honestly:

At work today, how many times did/have you washed your hands?

Count the number of times and write your answer here: _____

We will address this at the end of the chapter.

You know the old saying that you should "NEVER assume anything, as it makes an a$$ out of you and me"—well, when it comes to infection control, you should ALWAYS assume. What I mean by that is: ALWAYS assume that the patient you are working with is a carrier for infection!!

THE YUCKY STUFF

Let us begin by talking about the yucky stuff that can cause infections—those invisible little creatures in the air, on our bodies, and in the water that are always around us. Those microscopic little things are called microorganisms. Now, let's see if your office and/or work space contains any of the five elements that microorganisms need to grow and survive (Flynn, 2011, 2017).

1. Water
2. Food
3. Temperature
4. Light
5. Oxygen

My guess here is that your office does contain some if not all of these prerequisites that are needed for microorganisms to cultivate and live. Now think about your work space and all the objects that these living organisms can latch on to. Disgusting, right??

It's important to know that not all microorganisms cause infections, but the ones that do are known as pathogens. A pathogen is a tiny living organism that can make people sick. Pathogens are placed in three main categories: fungi, bacteria, and virus. So how do pathogens get into our offices and spread the likelihood of infection?

There are four main modes of transportation for microorganisms:

1. *Contact.* Contact transmission is the most common mode of transmission for microorganisms in a hearing aid dispensing practice and can be transmitted directly or indirectly. Every day you are extremely susceptible to this form of transmission just by the daily functions that you perform in your office. Direct contact can occur when you perform an otoscopic examination of a patient's ear with unwashed hands, where indirect contact can occur when you are handed a hearing aid from your patient and you handle that hearing aid with bare hands.
2. *Airborne.* Airborne transmission is where the pathogen is carried by air in the way of dust or moisture. These organisms can travel far and be widely dispersed by air until they land on a person who is susceptible.
3. *Vehicle.* Vehicle transmission refers to diseases transmitted by contaminated water, food, or objects.
4. *Vector borne.* Vector borne transmission is where a susceptible host is infected by an animal or insect that is carrying the pathogen. Regardless of the mode of transportation, the pathogen needs a way to enter our body, which is generally by our nose, eyes, skin, mouth, and, yes you guessed it, ears.

For your state licensing exam, it is imperative that you are aware of all forms of transmission, as it is expected that when you perform any direct or indirect process during your exam, you are following infection control protocols.

STANDARD PRECAUTIONS

Infection control is an important consideration for all health care providers who encounter patients both directly and indirectly. As hearing aid dispensers, you must be diligent in your practice to prevent the spread of disease. As a health care professional, you will handle many objects like hearing aids, earmolds, otoscope tips, ear impressions, headphones, ear inserts, etc. that can carry viruses, fungi, bacteria, and microorganisms. The Centers for Disease Control and Prevention (CDC) has developed guidelines and recommendations to minimize cross-contamination for health care workers. For these guidelines to be effective, it is important that YOU assume that every patient you encounter is a potential carrier of an infectious disease and that you take precautions.

The CDC has recognized hand washing as the single most important procedure for preventing the spread of infection. Hand washing can remove most pathogens just by using plain soap and water. Hands should be washed with hospital-grade antibacterial soap and water before and after every patient. If you do not have access to a sink in your office to wash your hands before and after every patient, antimicrobial "no rinse" hand sanitizers could also be used if they are used as directed.

Standard precautions are recommended by the CDC for the care of all patients regardless of whether they are known to be infected or not. Standard precautions are designed to reduce the spread of infection and apply to blood, non-intact skin, and all bodily fluid secretions and excretions, including cerumen and mucous membranes (OHSAH, 2008). Standard precautions include the use of hand hygiene, isolation precautions, appropriate personal protection

equipment such as gloves and masks, needle safety and sharps procedure disposal, as well as infectious waste disposal.

Hand Hygiene

Hand hygiene is considered the first line of defense and the most effective way to prevent the spread of infectious agents. It is the most important work practice and should be taken very seriously. Hand washing is especially taken seriously by your state on your licensing exam, especially for those who are working with real patients or subjects and when handling hearing aids, ear impressions, etc.

When to Wash Your Hands

1. Wash hands immediately before and after each patient.
2. Wash hands before and after situations where you are handling hearing aids, impressions, earmolds, etc.
3. Wash hands before and after removing and handling ear impressions.
4. Wash hands immediately after the removal of gloves.

How to Wash Your Hands

1. Make sure you have paper towels available before you begin to wash your hands. Paper towels are recommended over hand towels as they are for one-time use and can be thrown away afterward. The use of hand towels, unless used by only one person for one-time use, can cause contamination and the further spread of germs.
2. Turn on the water. Warm water is recommended.
3. Wet hands and apply soap. Liquid soap is preferred over bar soap, as bar soap can be a breeding ground for germs.

4. Once soap is applied, rub and scrub hands vigorously for at least 15 seconds.
5. While the water is still running, dry your hands with a paper towel and then use that towel to turn off the water. This prevents you from contaminating your clean hands.
6. Dispose of the towel.

If a sink is not readily available which will more than likely be the case when taking your state exam, an antimicrobial alcohol-based hand sanitizer rub can be used. Use an appropriate amount of sanitizer and rub hands together, making sure to rub in-between your fingers as well. Continue to rub until all the sanitizer is dry and do not use a towel to dry your hands. The use of hand sanitizers does not and should not take the place of hand washing using soap and water.

Personal Barriers

Gloves should be worn anytime you risk exposure to bodily fluids such as cerumen. Gloves should be worn when:

1. Handling hearing aids or earmolds directly from the patient
2. When there is visible drainage from the ear, blood, sores, or any type of lesion on the head
3. When cleaning and disinfecting instruments that may have been contaminated with cerumen
4. When handling probe tips, otoscope tips, or ear inserts
5. When removing or handling ear impressions
6. When performing cerumen management
7. When cleaning up contaminated areas
8. When handling dirty laundry
9. When working with a patient who is known to be immunocompromised

Gloves should not be reused, and they should be taken off immediately after use and thrown away. If you are using gloves, you should follow the proper procedure for removal of gloves, which is as follows:

1. When both hands are gloved, grab the outside of one glove at the top of the wrist.
2. Peel the glove off away from the body, turning the glove inside out.
3. Hold the removed glove in the hand that is still gloved.
4. With the ungloved hand, peel off the other glove by inserting your fingers inside of the glove at the top of the wrist.
5. Turn the second glove inside out and away from the body, leaving the first glove inside of the second.

Protective apparel must be worn when performing procedures that may expose one to infectious substances. Barriers such as gloves, eye protection, gowns, and disposable masks are to be worn when you may be at risk of the splash and splatter of infectious material and airborne contamination. For example, if it is within your scope of practice to perform cerumen removal by irrigation, ALL barriers should be worn. When handling hearing instruments and earmolds, especially when modifications are needed with grinding and buffing, masks and safety glasses are a must to reduce particles and microorganisms from getting in your eyes or being inhaled.

Cleaning, Disinfecting, and Sterilizing

The most important thing to know with cleaning, disinfecting, and sterilizing is they are NOT one and the same. They are in fact very different, and the process for each serves a different purpose. Cleaning is a process of removing visible gross contaminants from a surface, preparing that surface to be disinfected. Cleaning does not remove and kill germs! Disinfecting is the process of killing most germs by using a chemical solution to

Table 4–1. The Spaulding Classification (Courtesy of Suzanne Krumenacker)

Category	Level of Processing / Reprocessing	Examples
Non-Critical		
>These are considered items that do not directly come in contact with the patient or make contact with skin that is intact	Cleaning followed by the use of a Low Level Disinfectant (LLD)	Listening stethoscope, bone oscillator, headphones, patient response button, insert earphones.
Semi-Critical		
> Items that come in contact with cerumen because they can come into contact with blood and bodily fluids	Single use is preferred/ Sterilization or Disposable Cleaning followed by High Level Disinfection (HLD) as a minimum	Any item that enters the ear canal: Probe tips, otoscope tips, insert headphones, cerumen removal equipment, and probe tubes
> Items that come in contact with but do not penetrate non-intact skin or mucous membranes		
Critical		
> Items that directly enter the vascular system or sterile tissue	Cleaning followed by sterilization	Not applicable to hearing aid dispensing practice

do so. Environmental Protection Agency–approved hospital-grade disinfectants should be used in all dispensing practices. "In contrast to disinfecting, sterilization means killing 100 percent of the vegetative microorganisms and their endospores 100 percent of the time" (Kemp & Bankaitis, 2000).

It is important to know when it is acceptable to disinfect as opposed to sterilize. Items that do not encounter infectious substances or blood can be cleaned first and then disinfected. There is a guideline, known as the "Spaulding Classification," that was created to determine appropriate methods for reusing medical devices. This classification was created for any profession that it is based on the medical instruments intended use (Kennamer, 2007). According to the Spaulding Classification, these items would include headphones, earmolds, hearing aids, and surfaces that are not contaminated with visible contaminants such as blood and cerumen. Table 4–1 describes the Spaulding Classification and how it can be implemented into a hearing aid dispensing practice.

Infectious Waste Disposal

Although your state licensing exam may not be testing you directly on your knowledge of waste disposal, it is extremely important to know about the guidelines for proper waste disposal. This includes collecting, storing, decontaminating, and disposing of waste that is infectious and/or non-infectious, which is generally determined in accordance with state and federal regulations. Be sure to know what your state, as well as federal, regulations are before sitting for your exam. It is important to know that items that are disposable, such as otoscope tips and insert ear phones, can be disposed of in the regular trash. The only time this is not the case is if there is a significant amount of blood, cerumen, or ear drainage. If significant amounts do occur, then those items that are contaminated should be placed in a separate impermeable bag and labeled with the biohazard symbol. The bag should then be disposed of separately so that there is no chance of casual contact by you or anyone else in your office.

The other part to waste disposal includes sharp objects. Although we do not use needles in our practice, other instruments like razors should be disposed of in a "sharps container" or puncture-proof box. These items require a licensed waste disposal company to handle and dispose of them.

VERY INTERESTING (AND DISTURBING) STUDIES

The following information is probably not going to be on your state exam, but it is information that I personally believe to be eye opening to anyone getting into the field of hearing aid dispensing. I have included it in the reference section as well as on the companion website and encourage everyone to read both studies as soon as possible.

Remember the question that I asked you at the beginning of the chapter? I believe that by reading this chapter and getting a basic education on infection control, tomorrow your answer to that question will be different.

CONCLUSION

It is my hope that this chapter has shined some light on the topic and importance of infection control. For this book we just skimmed the surface on this topic so that you could know just enough to sit for your exam. I can't stress enough the importance

of reviewing your state website to see what the state's expectations are of you when it comes to your practical exam and infection control. In many states you will be performing tasks in which cross-contamination is a possibility, as many of you will be working with live subjects who are to be treated as if they were your patients.

In the "Putting It All Together" section for each module, I will refer to Standard Precautions a great deal, so it is extremely important that you follow these precautions to ensure that you are preventing the spread of infectious disease. Know that your state will be watching for this and may very well stop you from performing a task if you are at risk of cross-contamination which may affect the health and safely of everyone involved. The best way to be prepared for your exam is to make sure that you are following Standard Precautions in your office every day. If you are, then this topic should be second nature to you by the time you sit for your exam and the issue of cross-contamination will not even be a factor.

WHERE TO FIND MORE INFORMATION

https://www.cdc.gov/mmwr/PDF/rr/rr5116
.pdf
https://www.cdc.gov/infectioncontrol/pdf
/guidelines/disinfection-guidelines.pdf
https://www.fda.gov/
http://www.who.int/csr/bioriskreduction
/infection_control/en/
http://www.ihi.org/resources/Pages/Tools
/HowtoGuideImprovingHandHygiene.aspx

REFERENCES

Amlani, A. M. (1999). Current trends and future needs for practices in audiologic infection control. *Journal of the American Academy of Audiology, 10*(3), 151–159.

Burco, A. (2007). Current infection control trends in audiology, Paper 287 (Independent Studies and Capstones). http://digital commons.wustl.edu/cgi/viewcontent.cgi?article=1277&context=pacs_capstons

Burco, A. (2007). *Current infection control trends in audiology*. Unpublished AuD Capstone Project, Washington University. http://dspace.wustl.edu:8080/handle/1838/571

Flynn, L. (2011, 2017). *All about infection control*. Guelph, ON, Canada: Mediscript Communications Inc.

Kemp, R. J., & Bankaitis, A. E. (2000). *Infection control in audiology*. Retrieved from http://www.audiologyonline.com/articles/infection-control-in-audiology-1299

Kemp, R. J., & Bankaitis, A. E. (2000a). Infection control for audiologists. In H. Hosford-Dunn, R. Roeser, & M. Valente (Eds.), *Audiology diagnosis, treatment, and practice management* (vol. III, pp. 257–279). New York, NY: Thieme Publishing Group.

Kemp, R. J., & Bankaitis, A. E. (2000b). The germination of infection control in the audiology clinic. *The Audiology Journal*

Kemp, R. J., & Bankaitis, A. E. (2003). *Infection control in the hearing aid clinic*. Chesterfield, MO: Oaktree Products, Inc.

Kennamer, M. (2007). *Basic infection control for health care providers* (2nd ed.). Clifton Park, NY: Thomson Delmar Learning.

OHSAH (Occupational Health and Safety Agency for Healthcare in British Columbia). (2008). *Home and community care risk assessment tool: Resource guide*. http://www.phsa.ca/Documents/Occupational-Health-Safety/GuideHomeandCommunityCareRiskAssessmentToolResourc.pdf

⑤
Otoscopic Inspection

Objectives

- To prepare the candidate to perform a proper otoscopic examination
- To ensure that the candidate is taking hygienic precautions
- To ensure that the candidate is aware of FDA precautions

TERMS AND DEFINITIONS

Aseptic technique: a procedure to be performed under sterile conditions

Bridge-and-brace technique: a safety technique for holding equipment when used on a patient. Both hands need to be touching and act as one, as the equipment being used rests somewhere on the two hands. When approaching the patient, both hands and the equipment act as one and you rest your hands firmly on the patient's head.

Otoscope: an instrument used to visually examine the external ear canal and the tympanic membrane

Otoscopy: the process of examining the external ear canal and the tympanic membrane with an otoscope

Please refer to the glossary at the end of this book for more terms and definitions.

EQUIPMENT

The equipment that is used for performing an otoscopic examination on the state practical examinations consists only of a hand-held otoscope and speculums, as seen in Figure 5–1; portable video otoscopes are rarely permitted. Hand-held otoscopes can be battery operated, and those batteries are either rechargeable or replaceable. Such otoscopes come in many different sizes and can range in cost as well. It is recommended

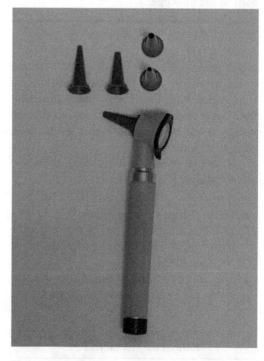

Figure 5–1. Typical otoscope along with several different sizes of speculums.

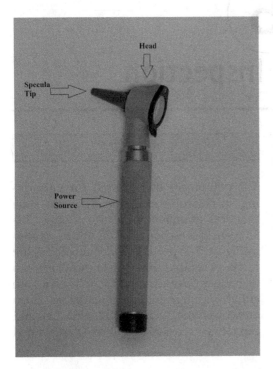

Figure 5–2. Portable hand-held otoscope and parts of the otoscope.

when purchasing or choosing an otoscope to be used for your practical examination that you ensure that it is reliable and that you have been able to practice with it so that you are 100% comfortable using it on the day of your exam.

The features of a hand-held otoscope are as follows (Figure 5–2):

1. Head (surgical, diagnostic)
2. Power source (standard or rechargeable batteries, 2.5-V incandescent or 3.5-V halogen bulb)
3. Specula (several sizes, reusable or throwaway, use largest without discomfort)

ASEPTIC TECHNIQUE

During the otoscopic examination, we must always have the patient's safety and comfort first and foremost in our minds. This is particularly important when we consider the possibility of cross-contamination, as discussed in the previous chapter. Unless proper precautions are followed, this could occur from one ear to another, from one patient to another, and lastly from patient to dispenser.

The following procedures have been designed to maintain a consistently high level of sterility for your equipment, and must be viewed as an essential part of your day-to-day routine.

1. Wash hands thoroughly before contact with the patient and your equipment.
2. Sterilize all equipment before using it on the patient.
3. Ensure that all of your equipment is placed on a sterile towel or surface.
4. Use gloves when handling the specula tips. If gloves are not accessible, use a sanitary wipe.
5. Only use one speculum tip per ear to avoid cross-contamination.
6. Always have extra sanitized specula on hand, if needed.
7. Dispose of speculum tip after use.
8. Wash hands.

The first step in your otoscopic examination of the patient should always be a thorough inspection of the outer ear. The reason for this is that the condition of the outer ear (including the back of the pinna) is of the utmost importance when considering the results of your audiometric test, in determining when to refer or not to refer the patient for a medical evaluation, in selecting the appropriate amplification for the patient, and lastly, for impression taking. Figure 5–3 is an example of a normal adult pinna.

When performing an otoscopic evaluation you should always check for the following:

1. *General condition of the ear canal.* In order to achieve a good impression, one must consider the size, shape, and texture

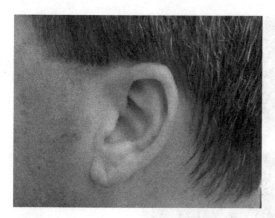

Figure 5–3. Example of a normal adult pinna.

(soft, medium, or hard) of the ear canal. Size and shape are important when taking an impression to decide which cotton otoblock to use. Texture is also important because you need to be aware of the amount of pressure you are using, because if the ear is a soft texture, the ear can be misshapen, causing a poor-fitting hearing aid. During the audiometric assessment, the condition of the ear canal can dictate whether or not you can proceed with your evaluation. For example, if one ear is impacted with cerumen, it will cause incorrect thresholds and, in turn, produce an inaccurate result.

2. *Obstruction.* It is usually caused by impacted or excessive cerumen, but could also be a foreign body (i.e., bug or cotton) as well. If the tympanic membrane is not visible, a conductive component to the hearing loss may be caused by the obstruction. Taking an ear impression on an ear that is obstructed may be painful, and even harmful, to your patient and therefore is not recommended. Refer the patient to a medical doctor.

3. *Discharge and/or drainage.* Any fluid in the canal can be classified as discharge and may sometimes be accompanied by a harsh odor. Fluid in the ear canal may be a sign of infection, and the patient should be referred to a medical doctor.

INSPECTING THE EAR CANAL

The following steps are provided to assist you regarding how to perform an otoscopic examination during your state licensing exam. Whether it is for impression taking or audiometric testing, the same steps should be taken.

- Use the proper bridge-and-brace technique for both left and right hands (Figures 5–4 A–C).
- Demonstrate a clean and safe procedure for inspecting the ear structures.
- Make sure to clean your otoscope speculum prior to touching it to the patient's ear.
- Describe the entire outer ear, including the back of the pinna.
- Look for foreign objects, excessive wax, abnormal growths, and so forth.
- Describe the ear canal.
- State whether or not the visual inspection allows you to proceed with the next task.

Here are the steps for using the otoscope correctly:

1. Attach the otoscope head onto the otoscope power base.
2. Find the largest speculum which will allow you to see into the ear canal. Using an alcohol wipe or sanitary cloth, clean the speculum and then gently twist it onto the narrow end of the otoscope head in a clockwise direction.
3. Turn the otoscope on by pressing the colored button and turning the otoscope head clockwise.
4. Hold the otoscope in your dominant hand with power base up, much like holding a pencil. Hold the otoscope close to the otoscope head, with thumb and first two fingers. Cushion the head with the heel of your hand to prevent trauma if the patient moves (see Figure 5–4).

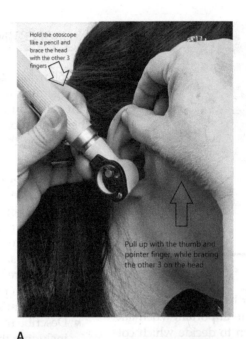

Hold the otoscope like a pencil and brace the head with the other 3 fingers

Pull up with the thumb and pointer finger, while bracing the other 3 on the head

A

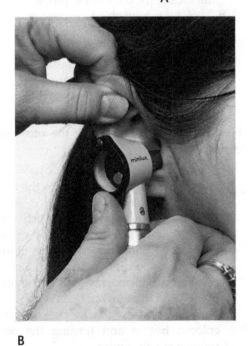

B

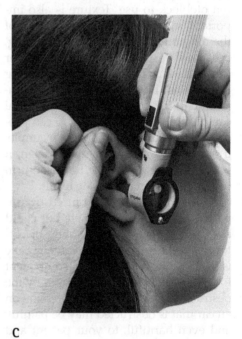

C

Figure 5–4. A. Example of the bridge-and-brace technique for left hand. **B.** Example of bridge and brace technique for the right hand. Follow the same instructions as with Figure 5–4A. **C.** Example of bridge-and-brace technique for the right hand. Follow the same instructions as with Figure 5–4A.

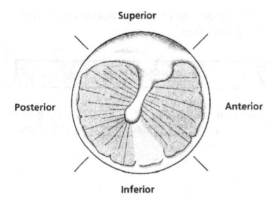

Figure 5–5. A healthy right eardrum. Note the "cone of light" in the 5 o'clock position. (From Taylor & Mueller, 2011, p. 50)

5. Watch carefully as you gently insert the speculum into the external canal. Stop when the speculum is 0.125 to 0.25 inch into the canal.
6. Look into the magnifying lens and through the speculum. You should be able to visualize the external canal and tympanic membrane, and the cone of light, as well as any cerumen or other obstacles. (See Figure 5–5 for the landmarks of the tympanic membrane.)

OTOSCOPIC INSPECTION FOR THE STATE EXAM

Prior to performing an otoscopic examination, you must ensure that the equipment has been properly sanitized as discussed previously, and that you have laid out your equipment on a sanitary surface, preferably a clean white towel.

1. Ensure that you have already asked your patient the FDA questions as discussed in Chapter 3, and that the answer to all of the questions is "No."

2. Prior to inspecting the ear, instruct the patient on what you are about to do. Your instructions can be anything that you are comfortable with as long as you are preparing the patient for the otoscopic exam. The following is an example of what you could say to instruct the patient: "What we are going to do is, I am going to take a look in your ears with my otoscope [show them the otoscope]. I will first be inspecting your right ear and then your left ear by checking outside and behind your ear first and then by looking inside your ear. It may feel a little uncomfortable but should not hurt. Just hold still while I inspect your ear and I will let you know when I am done. Do you have any questions before I begin?"
3. You can begin by washing your hands with a sanitary wipe, and then put the speculum tip on the otoscope, ensuring that there is no contact with the tip by using a sanitary wipe to fit the speculum.
4. Turn on the otoscope and visually check the outer ear and mastoid process behind the ear to ensure that there are no physical abnormalities.
5. Using the proper bridge-and-brace technique, insert the tip of the speculum carefully into the patient's ear canal, describing out loud what you are seeing. For example: "I see the first bend, I see the second bend, and I see the cone of light shining back at me. The ear canal is clear of debris and I can proceed with the testing and/or impression."
6. Using a sanitary wipe, remove the used speculum and throw it away. Using a clean sanitary wipe, fit another clean speculum tip to the otoscope and repeat steps 5 and 6 on the other ear.

It is important to note that all state examinations are not alike, and some may not even require you to perform an otoscopic examination on a real human ear. Consult your state information prior to the exam to know what is expected of you. If you are required to bring a human subject, before sitting for your practical examination, practice as much as you possibly can on as many ears as you possibly can to ensure that you are confident in the process of the procedure. Make sure that the subject you bring to the exam has healthy, normal ears with no obstruction.

REFERENCE

Taylor, B., & Mueller, H. G. (2011). *Fitting and dispensing hearing aids*. San Diego, CA: Plural Publishing.

6

Testing Equipment

WHAT IS A BIOLOGIC CHECK?

Performing a biologic check of your audiometer is an important step in your daily routine in your practice and is also a requirement on most state exams. A biologic check of the audiometric equipment refers to checking the instrumentation by biologic means, which in this instance includes determining the functionality of the equipment by listening to the equipment (DeRuiter & Ramachandran, 2010, p. 71). Check with your state prior to your exam to determine if they require your audiometer to be calibrated to ANSI standards (2004) and if a calibration sticker is required on your audiometer. You may also need to present documentation or a certification sheet that your audiometer has been calibrated in the past year at the time of your examination. Some states may only allow you to use headphones for testing, which means insert earphones are not permitted. If that is the case, make sure that your audiometer is calibrated with the headphones. Also important to note is whether or not the state requires a dual-channel versus single-channel audiometer and if there are any other specific guidelines that it may want you to follow.

The testing procedures required by your state determine what pieces of your audiometer will need to be accessed during your biologic check. Some states do not require you to perform speech testing, so in that instance, you will only need to verify the integrity of the headphones, inserts (if the state permits), and bone oscillator. For states that require speech testing, you must check the talkback system and monitored live voice or CD player to confirm that they are functioning properly.

HOW TO PERFORM A BIOLOGIC CHECK

In most instances for the state exam, you will be performing the biologic check on your own audiometer without the help of another individual. Upon completing your check, the proctors will perform their own biologic check once yours is complete to ensure that the equipment is functioning properly before you begin your audiometric testing. I highly recommend that you become very comfortable with the audiometer that you will be bringing to the exam, and that you are comfortable with performing the biologic check. It is generally part of the timed portion of your exam and you do not want to waste valuable time performing this check. Below are two examples of how you can perform the biologic check for your state exam based on the audiometric testing that you will be required to do.

Example 1

For states that require *only* pure-tone air and bone conduction testing and masking, do the following:

1. Wash your hands before beginning.
2. Open up your audiometer and plug it into the outlet.
3. Turn on the audiometer.
4. Remove the headphones and place them on the table. Ensure that the cords are untangled and free of knots.
5. Remove the bone oscillator and place it on the table. Ensure that the cords are untangled and free of knots.
6. Make sure that your cords and jacks are all plugged into the proper outlets. (Label them on your audiometer if you are not able to leave them plugged in so that you can quickly and effectively plug them into their proper places the day of your exam.)
7. Wash your hands before going any further.
8. Lay out a white towel, which will be your sanitary area for placing your sterile equipment.
9. Take a sanitary cloth and thoroughly wipe down the headphones and place them on the white towel.
10. Take a sanitary cloth and thoroughly wipe down the bone oscillator and place it on the white towel.
11. With a sanitary cloth, wipe down the face of the audiometer, including all knobs and buttons.
12. First test the headphones by placing them on your head and, starting with the right ear, choose a continuous tone on the audiometer and set the frequency dial to 1000 Hz. While moving the cords around, be listening that there is no static or intermittency of the continuous tone.
13. Repeat step 12 at another frequency of your choice.

14. Repeat steps 12 and 13 on the left ear.
15. Using a pulsed tone, go back to the right ear at 1000 Hz and slowly increase the dB level to see if you can hear the attenuation of the machine and that there is no static. Slowly decrease the tone and listen, checking that the tone is clear, then move on to another frequency and repeat the same procedure.
16. Repeat step 15 on the left ear.
17. Test the masking noise that you will be using for your testing and ensure that it is coming through the proper headphone, making sure to test both the right and left earphone.
18. Once you have tested the headphones, you can remove them but *do not* place them on your sterile towel. Just lay them on the table and proceed to check the bone oscillator.
19. Place the bone oscillator on your head behind either ear on the mastoid process and repeat steps 12 and 15.
20. After you have checked both the headphones and bone oscillator, repeat the sanitary procedure.
21. Take a sanitary cloth and thoroughly wipe the headphones and place them on the white towel.
22. Take a sanitary cloth and thoroughly wipe the bone oscillator and place it on the white towel.
23. Wash your hands before going any further.

Example 2

For states that require pure-tone air and bone conduction testing, speech testing, and masking, do the following:

1. Wash your hands before beginning.
2. Open up your audiometer and plug it into the outlet.
3. Turn on the audiometer.
4. Remove the headphones and place them on the table. Ensure that the cords are untangled and free of knots.

5. Remove the bone oscillator and place it on the table. Ensure that the cords are untangled and free of knots.

6. Make sure that your cords and jacks are all plugged into the proper outlets. (Label them on your audiometer if you are not able to leave them plugged in so that you can quickly and effectively plug them into their proper places the day of your exam.)

7. Wash your hands before going any further.

8. Lay out a white towel that will be your sanitary area for placing your sterile equipment.

9. Take a sanitary cloth and thoroughly wipe the headphones and place them on the white towel.

10. Take a sanitary cloth and thoroughly wipe the bone oscillator and place it on the white towel.

11. With a sanitary cloth, wipe down the face of the audiometer, including all knobs and buttons.

12. First test the headphones by placing them on your ears and, starting with the right ear, choose a continuous tone on the audiometer and set the frequency dial to 1000 Hz. While moving the cords around, be listening that there is no static or intermittency of the continuous tone.

13. Repeat step 12 at another frequency of your choice.

14. Repeat steps 12 and 13 on the left ear.

15. Using a pulsed tone, go back to the right ear at 1000 Hz and slowly increase the decibel level to see if you can hear the attenuation of the machine and that there is no static. Slowly decrease the tone and listen, checking that the tone is clear, then move on to another frequency to repeat the same procedure.

16. Repeat step 15 on the left ear.

17. Test the masking noise that you will be using for your testing and ensure that it is coming through the proper headphone when you go between both the left and the right earphone.

18. Once you have tested the headphones, you can remove them but *do not* place them on your sterile towel. Just lay them on the table and proceed to check the bone oscillator.

19. Place the bone oscillator behind either ear on the mastoid process and repeat steps 12 and 15.

20. Take a sanitary cloth and thoroughly wipe the bone oscillator and place it on the white towel.

21. Put the headphone on and change to microphone on the audiometer and check your talk-back microphone as well as the UV meter to make sure they are functioning properly for monitored live voice.

22. If you are using a CD player or iPod for speech testing, check the iPod/player as well as the CD to ensure that it is functioning properly.

23. Take a sanitary cloth and thoroughly wipe the headphones and place them on the white towel.

REFERENCES

American National Standards Institute. (2004). *Specifications for audiometers (S3.6-2004)*. New York, NY: Acoustical Society of America.

DeRuiter, M., & Ramachandran, V. (2010). *Basic audiometry learning manual*. San Diego, CA: Plural Publishing.

7

Basic Tympanometry

Objectives

- To prepare the candidate to understand the importance of tympanometry
- To prepare the candidate to be able to perform tympanometry
- To prepare the candidate to be able to interpret different types of tympanograms and the pathologies associated with those tympanograms

TERMS AND DEFINITIONS

Acoustic impedance: the total opposition to the flow of acoustic energy to the middle ear

Admittance: the opposite of impedance; a measure of how much energy flows through the system

Compliance: the opposite of stiffness

Immittance: a term used to describe the measurements of impedance and admittance

Tympanogram: a graphic representation of the air pressure and compliance of the middle ear

Tympanometry: measures how much sound bounces back off the TM as air pressure changes in the outer ear

Please refer to the glossary at the end of this book for more terms and definitions.

WHAT TO KNOW FOR YOUR STATE!

Tympanometry is one of those areas that almost every state wants their candidates to be knowledgeable about, but not all states allow those that dispense hearing aids to perform the test. It is very important to know what your state requires of you for both the written and practical portions of the hearing aid dispensing exam. If tympanometry is within your scope of practice for your state, then the "Putting It All Together" at the end of this module applies to you. If performing tympanometry is not within your scope of practice for your state, then the "Putting It All Together" at the end of this module is information that is just "good to know." Even if this section is not on your practical exam, it is likely that you will be tested on this information for your written exam.

After performing your case history and otoscopic inspection of the ear, tympanometry is performed to tell us the status of the middle ear. Tympanometry can be used for screening purposes or as part of your test battery. Tympanometry is an important part of your audiologic test battery, as it allows you to have an objective measure of the middle ear system (DeRuiter & Ramachandran, 2017, p. 27). This test is the most efficient and effective way to evaluate the middle ear and obtain information very fast without the patient having to participate; you only need the patient's ear.

The equipment that is used to test tympanometry is known by many names, such as "middle ear analyzer," "immittance bridge," "admittance instrument," and "immittance instrument." Every middle ear analyzer is different and can vary from manufacturer to manufacturer. Just like an audiometer, this piece of equipment basically has all the same controls, parts, and measurements. Figure 7–1 shows examples of different middle ear analyzers. Figure 7–2 shows the basic immittance probe and components for performing tympanometry. Be familiar with what those standard features and terms are for this equipment in order to "run" tympanometry for your practical exam. If you are not required to bring your own middle ear analyzer, you should be able to "run" theirs. Know what your state requirements and its expectations are when it comes to your exam so that you are prepared.

WHY TYMPANOMETRY?

So why is tympanometry so important? Tympanometry is not a test of hearing sensitivity. It is a test that helps us determine the condition of the middle ear prior to per-

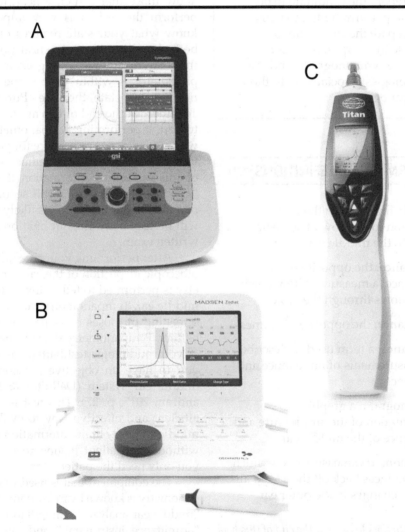

Figure 7–1. A few examples of middle ear analyzers. **A.** TympStar Pro from Grason-Stadler. **B.** Titan from Interacoustics. **C.** Zodiac from Madsen. (From Kramer & Brown, 2019, p. 214)

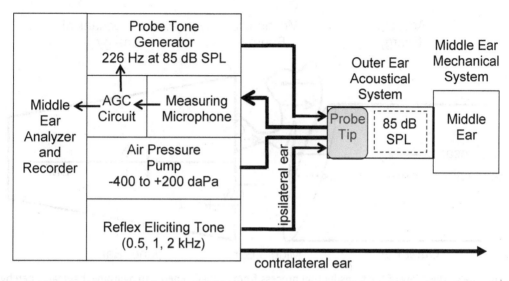

Figure 7–2. Block diagram showing the key components of a middle ear analyzer. (From Kramer & Brown, 2019, p. 215)

forming the hearing test. Tympanometry can give us a heads-up on what we might expect to see when we perform air and bone conduction testing and it will tell us if the patient needs to be referred for a medical evaluation. How does this test provide us with so much information about the middle ear? Tympanometry allows us to look at the ear as a mechanical system (McSpaden, 2006). To have a better understanding of this, let's tie it in to your pure-tone testing.

Let us first review how sound waves travel via air conduction. Sound collects in the outer ear and travels down the ear canal to the tympanic membrane (TM), which is considered *acoustic energy*. Those sound waves cause the tympanic membrane to vibrate and send those vibrations through the ossicular chain to the oval window, which is known as *mechanical energy*. A schematic of this is summarized in Figure 7–3. When the ossicles vibrate the oval window, it delivers the vibration to the fluid-filled cochlea via *hydromechanical energy*, which then causes the hair cells of the inner ear to cre-

ate nerve impulses, which are *electrical energy*. These impulses are then converted to *chemical energy* and processed in the brain. Refer to Table 7–1 for an explanation of the complete process.

To understand tympanometry, one must understand how the tympanic membrane acts when either positive or negative pressure is introduced into the external ear canal. For the TM to function most efficiently, pressure on both sides of it needs to be equal. Therefore, it is safe to say that when the pressure is not equal (positive or negative), a problem exists. Our ears function at atmospheric pressure (0 decapascal [daPa]). For clinical reasons we measure the middle ear function at greater or lesser pressures relative to ambient or atmospheric pressure (Hunter & Shahnaz, 2014). When we vary that pressure from positive to negative, immittance changes to the middle ear are seen and are shown graphically on the tympanogram.

Air conduction testing helps us to determine what the ear is actually doing by sending sound via air by way of headphones

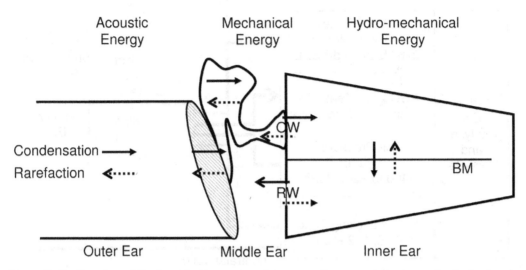

Figure 7–3. Overview of the transduction process from acoustic energy to hydromechanical, whereby the acoustic energy that enters the ear canal is converted to mechanical energy in the middle ear and then to hydromechanical energy in the inner ear. See Table 7–1 for further explanation. (From Kramer & Brown, 2019, p. 84)

or inserts, through the outer, middle, and inner ear. Bone conduction testing helps us to determine how efficiently the ear is sending sound through the bone directly to the cochlea by way of the bone oscillator, bypassing the outer and middle ear and determining what the ear can do. Now, after we have performed our pure tone testing and if the ear is functioning as well as it can with no air–bone gaps, we have determined that the type of hearing loss is sensorineural. If we have performed our pure tone testing and there is an air–bone gap present, we have then determined that a conductive component is present and there is some type of issue involving the mechanical system of the middle ear. Because tympanometry is not dependent on the person's hearing sensitivity and is only looking at the mechanical system of the ear, it is then possible to have a normal functioning mechanical system with no hearing sensitivity at all (dead ear).

For more on how the middle ear functions, check out the companion website.

TYMPANOMETRY

"Tympanometry measures how the admittance changes as a function of applied air pressure and how this function is affected by different conditions of the middle ear" (Kramer & Brown, 2019). The main assumption behind tympanometry is that in a normal middle ear, air pressure is EVEN on both sides of the tympanic membrane. When the pressures on both sides of the tympanic membrane are even, the TM will vibrate most efficiently and allow sounds to pass through it effectively. If the air pressure is NOT EVEN on both sides of the tympanic membrane, sounds will not pass through it efficiently or effectively and we have a problem (conductive component).

Tympanometry tests how much sound bounces back off the TM as air pressure changes in the outer ear. This procedure measures the movement of the eardrum as air pressure is increased or decreased in the

Table 7–1. Summary of the Auditory Transduction Processes (From Kramer & Brown, 2019, pp. 102–103)

Process	Part of Ear	Structures	Mechanism	Function
Acoustic	Outer	Auricle, ear canal	Resonance	Amplify mid to high frequencies to overcome impedance mismatch
Mechanical	Middle	Tympanic membrane, ossicles, oval window	Area, lever, and curved membrane advantages; route vibrations to oval window	Amplify low to mid frequencies to overcome impedance mismatch
Hydromechanical	Cochlea	Oval and round windows, scalae	Reciprocal in-and-out movements of oval and round windows	Instantaneous pressure variations in fluid-filled cochlea
		Basilar membrane	Passive process: traveling wave dependent on width and stiffness gradients of basilar membrane	Tonotopic place principle; highs at base and lows at apex; produces broad tuning curves
		Tectorial and basilar membranes, stereocilia	Bends stereocilia back and forth due to different pivot points of the two membranes; controls K+ flow into OHCs and IHCs	Activates hair cells: toward modiolus = excitation; away from modiolus = inhibition
Chemical-motoric	Cochlea	OHCs	Active process: OHC motility, from fluctuation in K+ flow, adds displacement to traveling wave to allow direct bending of IHC stereocilia	Increases sensitivity and sharpens tuning; responsible for sharp-tip region of tuning curves
Chemical-neural	Cochlea	IHCs	Increase and decrease of intracellular potential resulting from fluctuation in K+ flow	Controls release of neurotransmitter substance
Neural	8th Nerve	Auditory nerve fibers	Uptake of neurotransmitter substance; if adequate, cells initiate all-or-none discharges down 8th nerve axons to cells in cochlear nucleus	Neural discharge patterns provide intensity and frequency information to central nervous system

NOTE. IHC, inner hair cells; OHC, outer hair cells.

ear canal (dynamic compliance). Air pressure changes from positive to room air pressure to negative pressure. Normal findings are when the least amount of sound bounces back off the TM at room air pressure.

Measurement

To obtain a tympanogram, a probe is inserted into the ear canal ensuring a tight seal so that no sound can leak out. The probe consists of three holes, which include:

1. a tiny speaker that admits the tone into the ear canal
2. an air pump which is the way to change air pressure
3. a tiny microphone which picks up what sound is reflected off of the TM

Once a seal is made, pressure changes from positive to negative and a steady 226 Hz tone (aka probe tone) at 85 dB SPL is presented to the ear through the probe, shown in Figure 7–2.

When the air pressure changes from positive to negative:

- The probe speaker emits a tone.
- The probe mic picks up what bounces back off the TM.

Steps for obtaining a tympanogram:

1. Choose the appropriate size probe based on the patient ear canal size.
2. Insert probe into ear canal ensuring there is an air-tight seal.
3. Once the seal is made, a steady 226 Hz tone is presented at 85 dBSPL.
4. The air pump then adjusts the pressure equal to +200 daPa and at that time takes a measurement of the compliance.
5. As the pressure is increased, the tympanic membrane and ossicular chain stiffen due to the pressure.

6. At that time successive measurements are made of compliance as the pressure is decreased.
7. Once the pressure has reached 0 daPa or atmospheric pressure, negative pressure is created by the pump.
8. As the pressure changes occur, compliance measurements are made along the way (Figure 7–4).

DESCRIBING TYMPANOGRAMS

Just like we talked about in Chapters 1 and 2 about how to describe an audiogram by its three characteristics of type, degree, and configuration, a tympanogram is characterized by four measurements that help us to read and classify them. See Table 7–2. The four measurements are:

1. Physical volume (V_{ea})
2. Static compliance (Y_{tm})
3. Peak pressure (TPP)
4. Width (TW)

Physical Volume

Physical volume, which is also known as equivalent ear canal volume (ECV), "is a measurement of the volume of air in front of the probe in cubic centimeters (cc) or milliliters (mL) when the ear canal is pressured to +200 daPa" (DeRuiter & Ramachandran, 2017, p. 34). Measurement of equivalent ECV can be seen in Figure 7–5.

Static Compliance

Static compliance, which is also known as static admittance, is basically the height or peak of the tympanogram. Static compliance

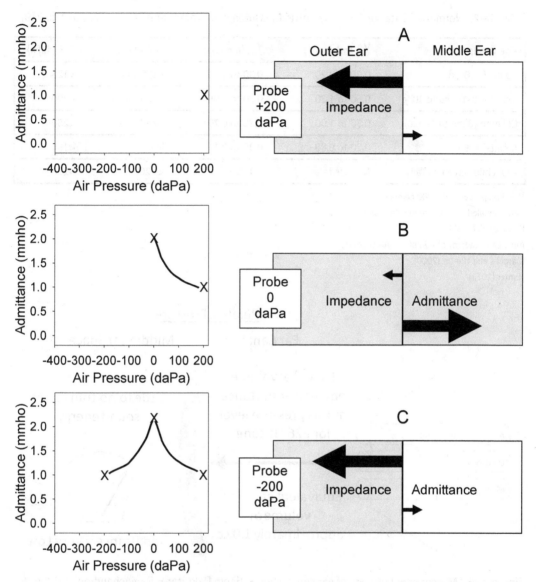

Figure 7–4. A–C. Illustration of how a normal tympanogram is generated. In A, the applied air pressure is at +200 daPa above atmospheric pressure and results in a minimum admittance that is equivalent to a relatively small cavity. This small admittance represents the admittance of only the outer ear because the tympanic membrane is not able to vibrate normally. In B, when the applied air pressure is lowered to 0 daPa (atmospheric pressure), the admittance reaches a maximum because the tympanic membrane can now vibrate most effectively. In this case, the admittance is equivalent to a larger cavity that represents the admittance of the outer and middle ear. In C, when the applied air pressure is at −200 daPa, the tympanic membrane does not vibrate effectively and the admittance is again equivalent to a small cavity that represents the admittance of only the outer ear. the actual admittance of the middle ear itself is represented by the difference between the maximum admittance and the admittance at +200 daPa.

Table 7–2. Normative Data for Tympanometric Measurement (From Kramer & Brown, 2019, p. 219)

Age Group	V_{ea} (mL or cc)	Y_{tm} (mmhos)	TPP (daPa)	TW (daPa)
Adults (>10 yr)	0.80 to 2.20	0.30 to 1.70	−105 to +5	<125
Children (>18 mo to 10 yr)	0.60 to 1.20	0.30 to 1.05	−75 to +25	<200
Children (6 mo to 18 mo)	0.50 to 1.00	0.20 to 0.70	−75 to +25	<250
Infants[1] (<6 mo)	0.20 to 0.80	0.40 to 2.10	NA	<150
AAA child screening fails	Not used	<0.20	<−200	>250

[1]1000 Hz probe tone; +200 compensation
Data compiled from the following sources:
Roush et al. (1995)
American Academy of Audiology [AAA] (2011)
Margolis and Hunter (2000)
Hunter (2013)

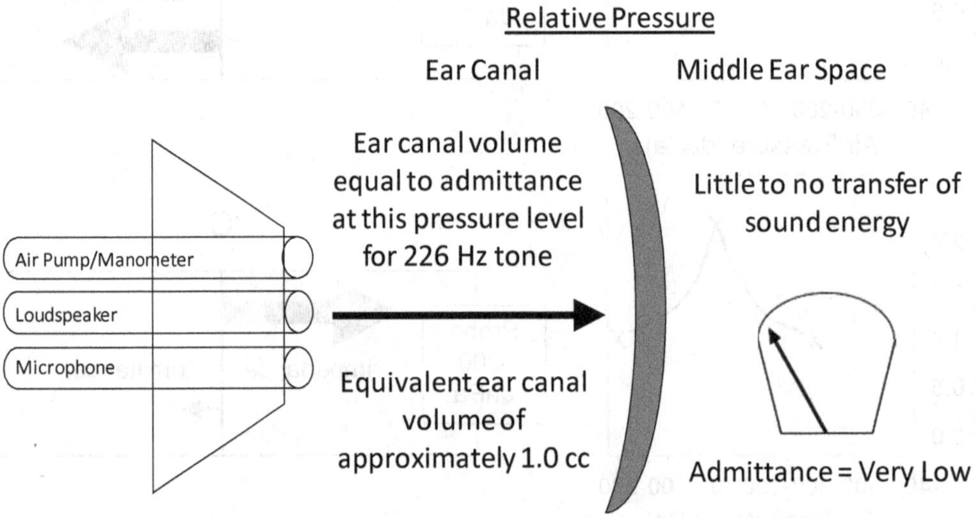

Relative Pressure

Ear Canal   Middle Ear Space

Air Pump/Manometer
Loudspeaker
Microphone

Ear canal volume equal to admittance at this pressure level for 226 Hz tone

Equivalent ear canal volume of approximately 1.0 cc

Little to no transfer of sound energy

Admittance = Very Low

Figure 7–5. Measurement process of ear canal volume. (From DeRuiter & Ramachandran, 2017, p. 34)

is measured in units of millimhos (mmho) or milliliters (mL). Figure 7–6 shows the measurement of static admittance.

- Tympanograms with normal compliance are known as Type A.
- Tympanograms with low static compliance are known as Type As.
  - s = shallow, short, or stiff

- Tympanograms with high static compliance are known as Type Ad.
  - d = deep

Peak Pressure

Peak pressure is the pressure at which the peak or static compliance occurs (Steiger &

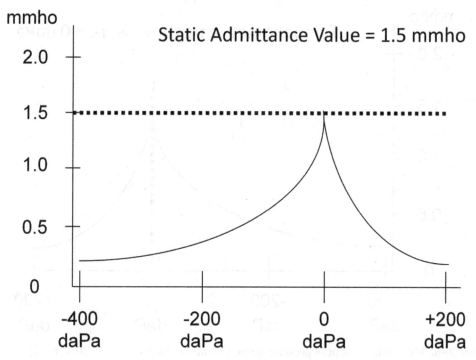

Figure 7–6. Measurement of static compliance. (From DeRuiter & Ramachandran, 2017, p. 33)

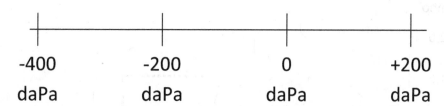

Figure 7–7. Range of ear canal pressure generated by the air pump. (From DeRuiter & Ramachandran, 2017, p. 31)

Miller, 2017). Peak pressure is identified in daPa and can be seen along the *x*-axis of the tympanogram, as seen in Figure 7–7. From this we can determine whether the pressure in the middle ear is positive or negative compared with the pressure of the ear canal. This measurement can be seen in the schematic in Figure 7–8.

- Tympanograms with no peak are known as Type B.

- Tympanograms with a peak pressure of −200 daPa or greater are known as Type C.

Width

Tympanogram width is a measurement in daPa at half of the static compliance of the peak to the compliance at +200 daPa. This measurement can be seen in Figure 7–9.

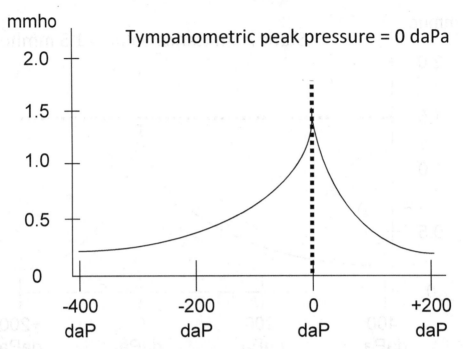

Figure 7–8. Measurement of peak pressure. (From DeRuiter & Ramachandran, 2017, p. 33)

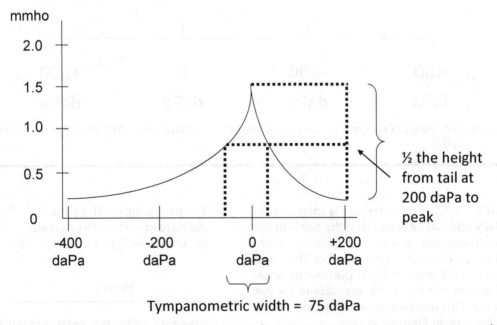

Figure 7–9. Measurement of tympanometric width. (From DeRuiter & Ramachandran, 2017, p. 34)

Table 7–3. Effects of Middle Ear Pathologies on Tympanometry (From Hunter & Shahnaz, 2014, p. 45)

	Admittance	TW	Volume	Mass	Springiness	Resonant Frequency
Middle ear effusion	Low	Wide	Normal	↑	↓	Low
Monomer/ossicular discontinuity	High	Narrow	Normal	↑	↑	Low
Perforation	Flat or variable	–	High	–	–	–
Tympanosclerosis	Normal to low	Normal	Normal	↑	↓	Low
Cholesteatoma	Low	Wide	Normal	↑	↓	Low
Lateral ossicular fixation	Low	Wide	Normal		↓	High
Medial ossicular fixation (otosclerosis)	Normal	Normal/narrow	Normal	–	↓	Normal to high

TW: tympanometric width.

Modified from Shanks (1984).

It is important to understand what the norms are for each of these measurements in order to know what the abnormal findings are and what they may represent in terms of disorders of the ear. It is important to note that assuming a pathology based solely on tympanometry is not recommended. Tympanometry should be performed as part of your test battery, and only then, when you have all the information, can a pathology be noted. Table 7–3 provides a delineation of the effects that middle ear pathologies can have on tympanometry.

TYMPANOGRAM TYPES

The shape or look of the tympanogram has long been the way a tympanogram has been classified based on the descriptions by James Jerger in 1970. The most widely used tympanogram shape types based on the four characteristics we just discussed are Type A, Type As, Type Ad, Type B, and Type C (shown in Figure 7–10).

- Type A as shown in Figure 7–10A has:
  - Normal peak height
  - Normal peak pressure
  - Normal ear canal volume
- Type B as shown in Figure 7–10B has:
  - No peak; it is flat.
  - Ear canal volume will be normal in cases of otitis media with effusion.
  - Ear canal volume will be large in cases where there is a perforation of the TM or in the case where pressure equalization tubes have been put in.
  - Ear canal volume will be low in cases of impacted cerumen or foreign bodies in the ear canal.
- Type C as shown in Figure 7–10C has:
  - Normal peak height, but reduced peak is also possible
  - Negative peak pressure
  - Normal ear canal volume

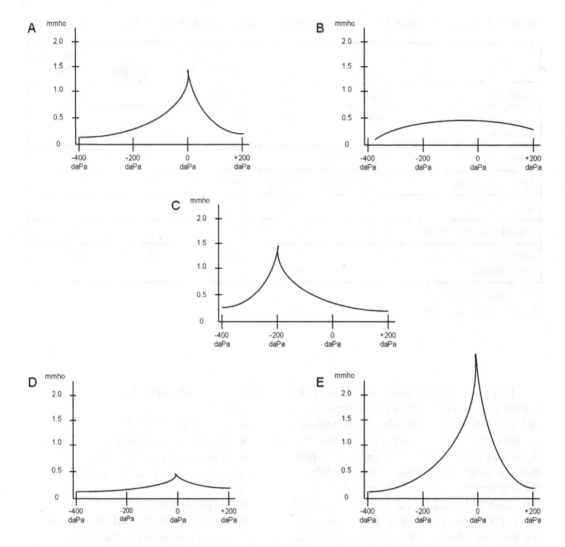

Figure 7–10. **A.** Type A tympanogram. **B.** Type B tympanogram. **C.** Type C tympanogram. **D.** Type As tympanogram. **E.** Type Ad tympanogram. (From DeRuiter & Ramachandran, 2017, p. 36)

- Type As as shown in Figure 7–10D has:
  - Abnormally low peak height
  - Normal peak pressure
  - Normal ear canal volume
- Type Ad as shown in Figure 7–10E has:
  - Abnormally high peak height
  - Normal peak pressure
  - Normal ear canal volume

CONCLUSION

Before performing a tympanogram on your test subject, I highly recommend performing one on your own ear. Get a feel for what is actually happening as you watch the tympanogram plotting on the screen. If you have a normal functioning middle ear, you will hear and feel the difference as the pressure goes from +200 daPa to 0 daPa to −300 daPa. You should be able to hear the change in the tone as the air pressure is increased or decreased. You should be able to hear the tone the loudest at the peak of the tympanogram where the admittance measurement is made that tells you how much energy flows through the system.

I hope this chapter helps you to perform, interpret, and understand the importance of tympanometry. Not only should this chapter assist with your state exam, but it should also serve as the basic building block for incorporating tympanometry into your test battery in your day-to-day practice (if it is within its scope). The references at the end of this chapter are a great resource if you are wanting more in-depth information about tympanograms.

REFERENCES

Clark, J. G., & Martin, F. N. (2009). *Introduction to audiology* (10th ed.). Boston, MA: Allyn and Bacon.

DeRuiter, M., & Ramachandran, V. (2017). *Basic audiometry learning manual* (2nd ed.). San Diego, CA: Plural Publishing.

Hunter, L. L., & Shahnaz, N. (2014). *Acoustic immittance measures*. San Diego, CA: Plural Publishing.

Jerger, J. (1970). Clinical experiences with impedance audiometry. *Archives of Otolaryngology, 92*, 311–324.

Kramer, S., & Brown, D. K. (2019). *Audiology: Science to practice* (3rd ed.). San Diego, CA: Plural Publishing.

McSpaden, J. B. (2006). Basic tympanometry in the dispensing office. *The Hearing Review, 13(12)*: 16–28.

Steiger, J., & Miller, E. L. (2017). *Diagnostic audiology: Pocket guide*. San Diego, CA: Plural Publishing.

8

Testing Procedures

Objectives

- To prepare the candidate to obtain unmasked air conduction thresholds
- To prepare the candidate to obtain unmasked bone conduction thresholds
- To prepare the candidate to obtain a speech reception threshold
- To prepare the candidate to obtain a speech discrimination score
- To prepare the candidate to obtain a most comfortable loudness level
- To prepare the candidate to obtain an uncomfortable loudness level

TERMS AND DEFINITIONS

Dynamic range: the difference between the speech reception threshold (SRT) and the uncomfortable loudness level (UCL) for speech

Monitored live voice (MLV): the presentation of a speech signal through a microphone on the audiometer. A volume unit (UV) meter on the audiometer is used to monitor the loudness of the signal.

Most comfortable level (MCL): the level that an individual feels is a comfortable level to listen to tones or speech

Phonetically balanced words: a list of monosyllabic words that are used to determine a person's speech discrimination score (SDS)

Pure-tone average (PTA): the average of thresholds in each ear at three frequencies: 500, 1000, and 2000 Hz

Speech discrimination score (SDS): the percentage of words that an individual repeats correctly when presented at a comfortable listening level

Speech reception threshold (SRT): the lowest level at which an individual can understand 50% of the time based on a list of spondee words

Spondee word: a word that consists of two syllables in which both syllables are presented with equal stress

Uncomfortable loudness level (UCL): the level at which a tone or speech becomes intolerable for an individual

Please refer to the glossary at the end of this book for more terms and definitions.

WHAT YOU NEED TO KNOW FOR YOUR STATE EXAM

Before we begin discussing the testing procedures, we first need to discuss what the states will be looking at and what you need to do to prepare yourself for your practical exam for this section. Read several times what the state provides you with as to what you are expected to do for the audiometric section of the practical exam. Every state is different, and with that being said, it is important that you not only know how to manually perform the battery of tests discussed in this manual, but that you can also verbally discuss the testing procedures. As discussed in previous chapters, you may need to bring your own audiometer or you may not need to bring one at all. States may provide you with an audiometer or simulator, so be prepared for what the state is testing you on and what its expectations are.

UNMASKED PURE-TONE AIR CONDUCTION TESTING

There are a few different techniques for testing procedures, but for the purpose of this manual, we will be looking at the most used techniques for the purpose of testing and fitting for hearing aids. The first test that you will be performing will be pure-tone air conduction testing. Before you begin, you would need to determine if the patient feels that he has a better ear and, if so, start audiometric testing on that side. If the patient is unsure, begin by testing the right ear. It is recommended to begin testing at 1000 Hz, as that is the frequency that is widely accepted as being the most easily heard by most individuals and it has been proven to be the most reliable with test/retest reliability (Carhart & Jerger, 1959).

Begin by using the ANSI recommended order for presentation, by testing 1000 Hz and then testing in ascending order to 2000, 4000, and 8000 Hz. Afterward, retest 1000 Hz on the first ear only (to ensure the patient understands the task), and then 500 and 250 Hz. In keeping with ASHA (1978) guidelines, begin by testing at a comfortable tone around 30 dB, unless there is a known hearing loss, in which case you would begin at 50 dB and then increase in 10 dB increments if there is no response to the initial presentation tone. To obtain a threshold, it is recommended that you use the modified Hughson–Westlake procedure (Hughson & Westlake, 1944), which consists of a descending and ascending technique (down 10 dB, up 5 dB) in order to obtain a valid and reliable threshold. The following is an example of how to perform the modified Hughson–Westlake procedure for obtaining an unmasked air conduction threshold at 1000 Hz. Visual representations for the steps below are given in Figure 8–1 to Figure 8–9:

- Present the tone at 30 dB: patient responds
- Decrease the tone (down 10) to 20 dB: patient responds
- Decrease the tone (down 10) to 10 dB: no response
- Increase the tone (up 5) to 15 dB: patient responds
- Decrease the tone (down 10) to 5 dB: no response
- Increase the tone (up 5) to 10 dB: patient responds
- Decrease the tone (down 10) to 0 dB: no response
- Increase the tone (up 5) to 5 dB: no response
- Increase the tone (up 5) to 10 dB: patient responds

So in this example, your threshold for this patient is 10 dB at 1000 Hz because the patient responded two-thirds of the time at 10 dB.

Step by Step

The following steps are for pure-tone air conduction testing using sanitary means for both you and your patient:

1. Wash your hands and seat the patient at a 90° angle away from the audiometer. This is done to prevent the patient from observing what you are doing on the audiometer and ensure that the patient is not getting any visual cues from you.

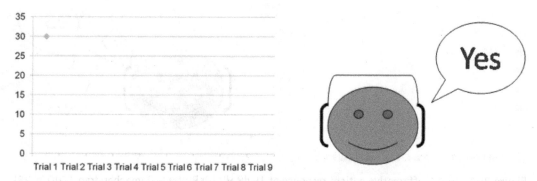

Figure 8–1. Trial 1: affirmative patient response at 30 dB HL. (From DeRuiter & Ramachandran, 2010, p. 77)

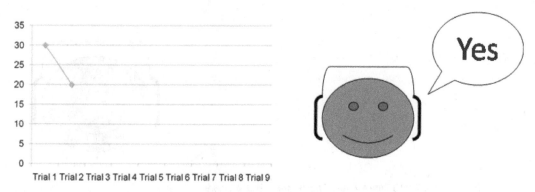

Figure 8–2. Trial 2: affirmative patient response at 20 dB HL. (From DeRuiter & Ramachandran, 2010, p. 77)

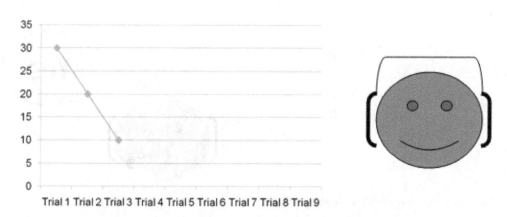

Figure 8–3. Trial 3: negative patient response at 10 dB HL. (From DeRuiter & Ramachandran, 2010, p. 77)

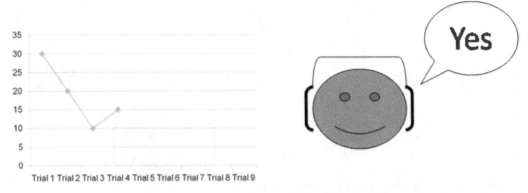

Figure 8–4. Trial 4: affirmative patient response at 15 dB HL. (DeRuiter & Ramachandran, 2010, p. 78)

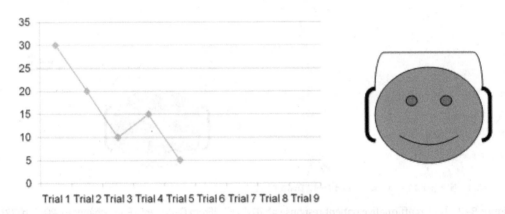

Figure 8–5. Trial 5: negative patient response at 5 dB HL. (From DeRuiter & Ramachandran, 2010, p. 78)

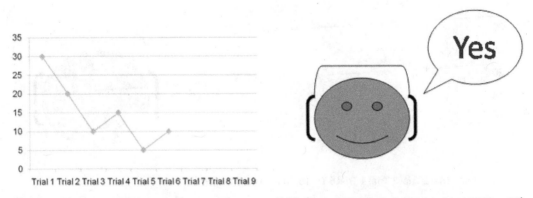

Figure 8–6. Trial 6: affirmative patient response at 10 dB HL. (From DeRuiter & Ramachandran, 2010, p. 78)

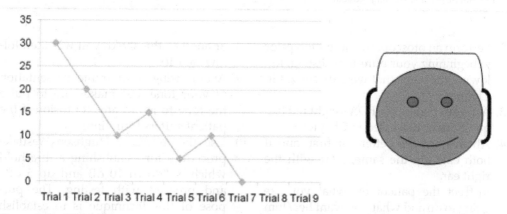

Figure 8–7. Trial 7: negative patient response at 0 dB HL. (From DeRuiter & Ramachandran, 2010, p. 79)

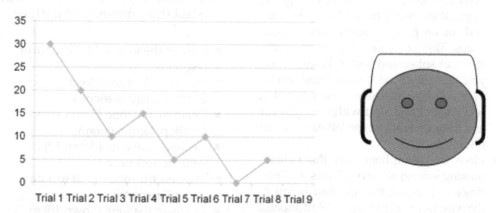

Figure 8–8. Trial 8: negative patient response at 5 dB HL. (From DeRuiter & Ramachandran, 2010, p. 79)

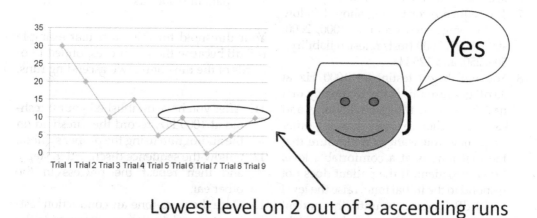

Lowest level on 2 out of 3 ascending runs

Figure 8–9. Trial 9: affirmative patient response at 10 dB HL. (From DeRuiter & Ramachandran, 2010, p. 80)

2. Perform an otoscopic examination prior to beginning your pure-tone testing, following the steps that were discussed in Chapter 5.
3. Ask your patient the FDA's eight red flag questions as discussed in Chapter 3.
4. Always test the better ear first, and if both ears are the same, start with the right ear.
5. Instruct the patient on what you are going to do and what you want her/him to do. Proper instruction is extremely important to make sure that you get the most accurate results. For example: "What we are going to do is, I am going to put these headphones over your ears and you are going to hear various tones/beeps. The tones will start off loud and then get softer and softer. What I want you to do is to raise your hand whenever you hear the tone even when it is really soft. I will start with the right ear and then we will test the left ear. Do you understand?"
6. Place the headphones on the patient, making sure to remove glasses and earrings and ensure that the hair is out of the way. If using traditional headphones, place the red headphone over the right ear and the blue headphone over the left ear, making sure to check for collapsed ear canals. Tighten the headband to ensure that it does not move.
7. The sequence for testing should follow ANSI's suggested order of 1000, 2000, 4000, 8000, 1000 (test/retest reliability), 500, 250, and 125 Hz.
8. You will begin testing at 1000 Hz at 30 dB because this is the frequency that has the best test/retest reliability and can be heard more easily than any other frequency. You want to make sure that the first tone is at a comfortable level for your patient. If the patient does not respond to the initial tone, raise the level in 10 dB increments until the patient elicits a response. Once you have established a response, whether it is at 30 dB

or another threshold, you will then follow step 10.
9. Avoid using a rhythmic presentation of your tone and make sure to pulse the tone to avoid any confusion if the patient suffers from tinnitus.
10. Use the modified Hughson–Westlake procedure for establishing a threshold which is "down 10 dB and up 5 dB" and proceed with testing. The purpose of this technique is to establish the patient's threshold. Threshold is the lowest level at which a patient can hear the tone two-thirds of the time when ascending. Below is an example of establishing threshold at 1000 Hz:

- Present the tone at 30 dB: patient responds
- Decrease the tone (down 10) to 20 dB: patient responds
- Decrease the tone (down 10) to 10 dB: patient responds
- Decrease the tone (down 10) to 0 dB: no response
- Increase the tone (up 5) to 5 dB: patient responds
- Decrease the tone (down 10) to –5 dB: no response
- Increase the tone (up 5) to 0 dB: no response
- Increase the tone (up 5) to 5 dB: patient responds

Your threshold for this particular example is 5 dB because the patient responded two-thirds of the time or on two ascending runs.

11. After you have established your threshold at 1000 Hz, record the threshold on the audiogram using the proper symbol.
12. Follow the sequence discussed in step 7 and then repeat the process in the other ear.
13. Once the pure-tone air conduction testing is complete, you can move on to the pure-tone bone conduction testing.

UNMASKED PURE-TONE BONE CONDUCTION TESTING

The purpose of bone conduction testing is that it helps to determine the cochlea's function and is the determining factor as to the type of loss that a patient has, as discussed in Chapter 2. Pure-tone bone conduction testing can take place at two different stages within the battery of tests. It can be tested right after pure-tone air conduction testing or after speech testing. For unmasked pure-tone bone conduction testing, the frequencies that are tested are different from those that are tested for air conduction testing, and are as follows: 250, 500, 1000, 2000, and 4000 Hz.

For the purpose of this manual, we present bone conduction testing after air conduction testing with the assumption that a hearing loss will be present in a majority of the patients you will be testing in your practice. It is a good habit to perform bone conduction testing after air conduction testing, especially when a hearing loss is present with air conduction thresholds.

Step by Step

The following steps are for pure-tone bone conduction testing using sanitary means for both you and your patient:

1. Wash your hands.
2. Remove the headphones from the patient's head and place them back on your sanitary surface.
3. Instruct the patient on what you are going to do and what you want him or her to do. Proper instruction is extremely important to make sure that you get the most accurate results. For example: "What we are going to do now is, I am going to put this device behind your ear and you are going to hear the vari-

ous tones/beeps again. The tones will start loud and then get softer and softer. What I want you to do is to raise your hand whenever you hear the tone, even when it is really soft. It does not matter which ear you hear the tones in; as long as you hear them, I would like you to raise your hand. Do you understand?"

4. Place the bone oscillator on the patient's head, directly behind the pinna on the mastoid process as seen in Figure 8–10. Ensure that the bone oscillator is not touching the patient's pinna and that all of the patient's hair is out of the way as well.
5. Begin by testing at 1000 Hz at 30 dB, same as you did for air conduction testing.
6. The sequence for testing should follow ANSI's suggested order of 1000, 2000, 4000, 500, and 250 Hz.
7. Avoid using a rhythmic presentation of your tone and make sure to pulse the tone to avoid any confusion if the patient suffers from tinnitus.
8. Use the modified Hughson–Westlake procedure for establishing threshold, which is "down 10 dB and up 5 dB" and proceed with testing. The purpose of this technique is to establish the patient's threshold. Threshold is the lowest level at which a patient can hear the tone

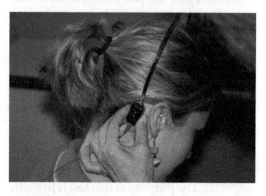

Figure 8–10. Bone conduction oscillator placement on a patient. (From Valente, 2009)

two-thirds of the time when ascending. Below is an example of establishing threshold at 1000 Hz:

- Present the tone at 30 dB: patient responds
- Decrease the tone (down 10) to 20 dB: patient responds
- Decrease the tone (down 10) to 10 dB: no response
- Increase the tone (up 5) to 15 dB: patient responds
- Decrease the tone (down 10) to 5dB: no response
- Increase the tone (up 5) to 10 dB: no response
- Increase the tone (up 5) to 15 dB: patient responds
- Decrease the tone (down 10) to 5 dB: no response
- Increase the tone (up 5) to 10 dB: no response
- Increase the tone (up 5) to 15 dB: patient responds

Your threshold for this particular example is 15 dB.

1. After you have established your threshold at 1000 Hz, record the threshold on the audiogram using the proper symbol.
2. Follow the sequence given in step 6 and then repeat the process in the other ear.
3. Once the pure-tone bone conduction testing is complete, you can move on to speech testing.

SPEECH RECEPTION THRESHOLD

Speech reception threshold can be defined as the lowest level at which the patient understands speech 50% of the time (Martin, 1991). The purpose of this test is to verify and check the reliability of your pure-tone testing and to ensure that the patient's SRT is within ±10 dB of the pure-tone average

Table 8–1. One List of Spondee Words from CID W-1 Word List

Airplane	Eardrum	Iceberg	Railroad
Armchair	Farewell	Inkwell	Schoolboy
Baseball	Grandson	Mousetrap	Sidewalk
Birthday	Greyhound	Mushroom	Stairway
Cowboy	Hardware	Northwest	Sunset
Daybreak	Headlight	Oatmeal	Toothbrush
Doormat	Horseshoe	Padlock	Whitewash
Drawbridge	Hotdog	Pancake	Workshop
Duckpond	Hothouse	Playground	Woodwork

Source: Taylor and Mueller (2011).

(PTA). The PTA is determined by calculating the patient's thresholds at 500, 1000, and 2000 Hz, adding them together, and then dividing by three in each ear. (We discuss PTA more in depth later in this chapter.)

The following is a modified approach to the method that was set forth by ASHA (1988) and Martin and Downey (1986) for obtaining an SRT. The types of words that are used for SRT testing are known as spondee words. Spondee words are two-syllable words, such as playground and baseball, which have the same amount of stress and intensity on each syllable. Most state exams will have you verbally administer these words, so make sure that you practice so that you are able to present these words at 0 dB on the volume unit (VU) meter for each syllable. The Central Institute for the Deaf (CID) developed the spondee word list, which consists of 36 words (Table 8–1).

SPEECH AUDIOMETRY

After performing pure-tone testing, you can perform speech testing, of which there are several types; however, for the purpose of the hearing aid dispenser state licensing examinations, we cover only the following most commonly used types:

1. Speech reception threshold (SRT)
2. Speech discrimination (SD) / word recognition (WR)
3. Most comfortable level (MCL)
4. Uncomfortable level (UCL)

Step by Step

The following steps are for testing SRT using sanitary means for both you and your patient:

1. Wash your hands.
2. Remove the bone oscillator from the patient's head and place it back on your sanitary surface.
3. Instruct your patient as to what you are about to do. For example: "What we are going to do now is, I am going to present a list of words to you in each ear. The words will start off loud and then get softer and softer. What I would like you to do is repeat the word back to me as best you can. It is fine to take a guess if you must. We will start with your right ear and then test your left ear. Do you understand?"
4. Place the headphone on the patient's head.
5. First determine the patient's PTA based on the pure-tone thresholds and start your SRT testing 40 dB above the PTA. (If the threshold is not known, then start at 50 dB HL.)
6. Start by familiarizing the patient with the words at the starting level by saying approximately 10 words to get the patient comfortable.
7. In 10 dB descending steps, present one spondee word at a time. If the patient repeats it correctly, then decrease in 10 dB steps until the patient misses a word.
8. When the patient misses a word, increase the level 5 dB and present one spondee word. If the patient misses, then increase another 5 dB until the patient responds correctly.
9. Once you obtain a correct response, decrease in 10 dB increments and repeat steps 7 and 8.
10. When you have presented one spondee at each level and have obtained a correct response three times, this is considered your threshold.
11. Mark your SRT in the proper place on the audiogram.
12. Once you have obtained your threshold in the right ear, repeat steps 5 to 10 on the left ear.

Example of Obtaining an SRT

Let us assume that you obtained your pure-tone thresholds and now you need to determine the patient's PTA. Your thresholds in the right ear are 500 Hz = 0 dB, 1000 Hz = 10 dB, and 2000 Hz = 20 dB; and the thresholds in the left ear are 500 Hz = 15, 1000 Hz = 15, and 2000 Hz = 15. So when we calculate, the PTA in the right ear = 10 dB and the PTA in the left ear = 15 dB. If we follow the steps for determining SRT as previously discussed, we are going to take our PTA and add 40 dB, and that will be our starting point for our SRT testing. So in this example, our PTA in the right ear is 10 dB. We are going to add 40 dB and then begin our SRT testing in the right ear at 50 dB. The process is the same that we used for pure-tone testing as we will "decrease 10 dB" for correct responses and "increase 5 dB" for incorrect responses.

1. We begin presenting about 10 words to the patient's right ear at 50 dB to familiarize the patient with the list (baseball, ice cream, toothbrush, cowboy, iceberg, etc.), and then we decrease the words in 10 dB increments and present another word.
2. Present at 40 dB "hardware"—repeated correctly (decrease 10 dB)

3. Present at 30 dB "sunshine"—repeated correctly (decrease 10 dB)
4. Present at 20 dB "toothbrush"— repeated correctly (decrease 10 dB)
5. Present at 10 dB "cowboy"—incorrectly repeated (increase 5 dB)
6. Present at 15 dB "ice cream"—repeated correctly (decrease 10 dB)
7. Present at 5 dB "baseball"—incorrectly repeated (increase 5 dB)
8. Present at 10 dB "railroad"—incorrectly repeated (increase 5 dB)
9. Present at 15 dB "cowboy"—repeated correctly (decrease 10 dB)
10. Present at 5 dB "sunshine"—incorrectly repeated (increase 5 dB)
11. Present at 10 dB "iceberg"—incorrectly repeated (increase 5 dB)
12. Present at 15 dB "hardware"—repeated correctly (SRT = 15 dB)

You have obtained your SRT when the level is reached at which your patient has repeated the words correctly 50% of the time. In this example, our patient's PTA in the right ear is 10 dB and our SRT was obtained at 15 dB, which is within ±10 dB; thus, we can conclude that the results are reliable.

SPEECH DISCRIMINATION AND WORD RECOGNITION

Speech discrimination (SD) testing, also known as word recognition (WR) testing, can be defined as the number of correctly repeated words that are presented to the patient at slightly above UCL. The purpose of this test is:

1. To determine if there is a pathology in the auditory system
2. To determine the extent of a patient's understanding ability
3. To determine the need for amplification
4. To determine a game plan for aural rehabilitation

Both SD and WR testing are performed by presenting a list of 50 monosyllabic words that are phonetically balanced, meaning words that contain all of the phonetic elements in the English language (Martin, 1991, p. 132). There are many different weighted lists available to use, but for the purpose of this manual, we refer to the most widely used list in the United States, the Northwestern University List 6 (NU6), which can be found in Appendix B at the back of this book.

Since each list is 50 words, it is recommended that all 50 words be administered to achieve the most accurate WR score. For the sake of saving time, many people only administer 10 or 25 words, and since the lists are not made to be halved, this means the WR score is not truly a reliable and accurate score of the patient's discrimination ability because not all the phonemes were tested. For people who have to test WR or discuss WR testing on their state examination, this is very important to know. So best practices guidelines state that each patient should be presented 50 words in each ear and that each word be valued at 2% or 2 points for each word repeated correctly (Taylor & Mueller, 2011, p. 100).

There are two methods that can be used for the presentation of the stimulus, monitored live voice (MLV) and recorded. Since most state exams are testing to see that you know how to perform the audiometric tests, we discuss WR testing using MLV. So how do you determine the level at which to test for WR testing? A general practice among most licensed hearing aid dispensers is to present the list of 50 words at 40 dB above your SRT. The level for this test should be slightly louder than the MCL (discussed later in this chapter) for the patient.

Step by Step

The following steps are for the testing procedure to determine a patient word recognition/speech discrimination score:

1. Determine the level at which you are going to be presenting the word list.
2. Instruct your patient as to what you are going to do. For example: "What we are going to do now is, I am going to say some more words to you. This time the words will not get any softer; they are going to stay at one level. What I would like you to do is to repeat the word back to me as best you can. I will be presenting the words at the end of a phrase, I will say 'Say the word' and I would like you to only repeat the word to me at the end of the phrase as best you can, and you can take a guess if you have to, if you are unsure of the word you heard. Do you understand?"
3. Test starting with the patient's better ear, and if the hearing loss is symmetrical, start with the right ear.
4. Present the list of 50 words keeping track of every word that the patient repeats incorrectly.
5. After you have presented all 50 words, count the incorrect words (remember that each incorrect word is worth

2 points) and subtract by 100, and that is your SD score for that ear.
6. Mark your score in the appropriate area on your audiogram.
7. Repeat steps 1 to 6 on the opposite ear. (You can skip step 2, since you have already instructed the patient.)

MOST COMFORTABLE LEVEL

The purpose of testing a patient's MCL is to help to determine what level of speech will generally be comfortable to the patient, which is extremely important information when fitting hearing aids. For normal-hearing patients, their MCL is generally between 40 and 50 dB HL. For those patients who exhibit a hearing loss, that level may vary. Based on the patient's dynamic range, the MCL is about the halfway point between the SRT and the patient's uncomfortable loudness level (UCL). Figure 8–11 illustrates the difference seen in the dynamic

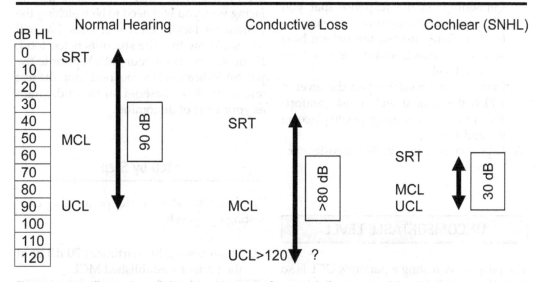

Figure 8–11. Illustration of the dynamic range for speech for a normal-hearing ear, a conductive hearing loss, and a cochlear hearing loss. The dynamic range for speech is the difference between the speech recognition threshold (SRT) and the uncomfortable loudness level (UCL). Most notable is the greatly reduced dynamic range (e.g., 30 dB) seen with cochlear hearing losses. (From Kramer, 2008)

range depending on the type of hearing loss that the patient exhibits.

Step by Step

The following steps are for performing MCL testing:

1. Testing is done by starting 40 dB above the SRT at about the same level at which you performed your SDS/WR testing.
2. Start with the better ear first, and if the loss is symmetrical, start with the right ear.
3. Instruct the patient on what you are going to do. For example: "What we are going to do now is, I am going to continually talk to you, and what I want to find out is the level at which it is most comfortable for you to listen to me. So at the level that my voice is at right now, listen to my voice while I count from 1 to 10; if I were a television and you had to listen to me, would you turn me up, turn me down, or leave me just where I am?" Then you count to 10.
4. Depending on the response that you get, you will increase or decrease the level by 5 dB and ask the patient how your voice sounds and if it is at a comfortable level.
5. Once you have established the level at which the patient feels most comfortable, mark it in the appropriate place on the audiogram.
6. Repeat steps 1 to 5 on the opposite ear.

UNCOMFORTABLE LEVEL

The purpose of testing a patient's UCL is so that when and if the patient is fit with hearing aids, it is imperative that you know at what level sounds become uncomfortable,

as you never want to exceed that level with hearing aids. A patient's UCL, also known as threshold of discomfort (TD) and loudness of discomfort level (LDL), can be defined as the level at which speech and/or tones become so uncomfortable that the patient could not tolerate it for any length of time.

Different from MCL testing, UCL testing can be performed either by testing speech in each ear, as is done for MCL testing, or by testing frequencies using tones. Since there are various ways that UCLs can be tested, check with the information provided by your state to determine which method you will need to perform and how the state wants you to perform it. If you are in a state in which you just need to describe and discuss the different audiometric tests, be aware of the two different ways in which UCL can be tested. One very important aspect with UCL testing that differs from the other audiometric tests is that you want the patient to face you while you are performing this test. The reason for this is that some people feel that they need to withstand louder speech or tones before actually reporting it to the hearing professional. Since the patient will be facing you, you will need to be watching the patient for facial gestures or cues that will let you know that the stimulus is too loud. If you see this from your patient prior to the patient indicating it is too loud, stop the test and mark that threshold on the audiogram as your level of discomfort.

Step by Step

The following steps are for performing UCL testing by speech:

1. Begin testing by starting at 70 dB or at the patient's established MCL.
2. Start with the better ear first, and if the loss is symmetrical, begin by testing the right ear first.

3. Instruct the patient on what you are going to do. For example: "What we are going to do now is, I am going to continue to talk to you and while I do, my voice will continue to get louder and louder. What I would like you to do is to listen to my voice and raise one finger when my voice becomes loud, and then when my voice becomes uncomfortably loud where you would not want to listen to it anymore, raise your whole hand and I will stop. So one finger for loud and whole hand for uncomfortably loud, and I will stop. Do you understand?"

4. Test by continually talking to the patient and raising the level of your voice slowly in 5 dB increments until the patient responds with the whole hand, you reach the limit of the audiometer, or you visually recognize that the patient is experiencing discomfort.

5. Mark the threshold in the appropriate place on your audiogram.

6. Repeat steps 1 to 5 on the opposite ear.

Step by Step

The following steps are for obtaining UCLs by tones at each frequency:

1. When testing UCL, tones by frequency are generally obtained in each ear at 500, 1000, 2000, and 4000 Hz.

2. Begin by testing the better ear; if the ears are symmetrical, start with the right ear.

3. Instruct the patient on what you are going to do. For example: "What we are doing to do now is I am going to present some tones to you. The tones will start off loud and continue to get louder and louder. What I would like you to do is to raise your finger when you feel that the tone is loud, and when you feel the tone is uncomfortably loud where you wouldn't want to listen to it anymore, raise your whole hand and I will stop. So

raise your finger for loud, and raise your whole hand for uncomfortably loud and I will stop. Do you understand?"

4. Begin at 70 dB HL or at the known level of MCL by tone at 1000 Hz, and present the tone by pulsing it in 5 dB increments until the patient responds by raising the whole hand, you reach the limit of the audiometer, or you visually recognize that the patient is experiencing discomfort.

5. Once you have obtained that response, mark it on the audiogram using the symbol provided in the legend on the correct frequency for UCL.

6. You will then continue testing at 2000, 4000, and 500 Hz, recording your findings.

7. Once you have completed testing on one ear, follow steps 4 to 6 on the opposite ear.

I hope this chapter helps you to understand and perform the basic hearing test battery needed to pass your state licensing exam. Not only will this chapter assist you in your studies, it is also essential for day-to-day testing in practice once you have passed your state exam. (Reminder: Make sure you practice testing on whomever you can get to ensure that you have this process down seamlessly.)

REFERENCES

American Speech-Language-Hearing Association (ASHA). (1978). Guidelines for manual pure-tone audiometry. *ASHA, 20*, 297–301.

American Speech-Language-Hearing Association (ASHA). (1988). Guidelines for determining the threshold level for speech. *ASHA, 30*, 85–89.

Carhart, R., & Jerger, J. F. (1959). Preferred method for clinical determination of puretone thresholds. *Journal of Speech and Hearing Disorders, 24*, 330–345.

DeRuiter, M., & Ramachandran, V. (2010). *Basic audiometry learning manual.* San Diego, CA: Plural Publishing.

Hughson, W., & Westlake, H. D. (1944). Manual for program outline for rehabilitation of aural casualties both military and civilian. *Transactions of the American Academy of Ophthalmology and Otolaryngology, 48*(Suppl.), 1–15.

Kramer, S. (2008). *Audiology: Science to practice* (p. 192). San Diego, CA: Plural Publishing.

Martin, F. N. (1991). *Introduction to audiology* (4th ed.). Englewood Cliffs, NJ: Prentice-Hall.

Martin, F. N., & Downy, L. K. (1986). A modified spondee threshold procedure. *Journal of Auditory Research, 26,* 115–119.

Taylor, B., & Mueller, H. G. (2011). *Fitting and dispensing hearing aids.* San Diego, CA: Plural Publishing.

Valente, M. (2009). *Pure-tone audiometry and masking* (p. 28). San Diego, CA: Plural Publishing.

9

Concepts of Masking

Objectives

- To ensure the candidate understands the concept of masking
- To prepare the candidate to recognize the need for masking
- To prepare the candidate to know why there is a need for masking
- To prepare the candidate to obtain masked air conduction thresholds
- To prepare the candidate to obtain masked bone conduction thresholds
- To prepare the candidate to obtain masked speech reception thresholds
- To prepare the candidate to obtain masked speech discrimination scores

TERMS AND DEFINITIONS

Effective masking (EM): the minimum amount of masking noise that is required to just mask out a signal

Interaural attenuation (IA): the loss of acoustic (sound) energy of a sound as it travels from the test ear across to the opposite ear

Masking: the process by which a noise is introduced to the nontest ear to prevent that ear from responding when testing the opposite ear

Nontest ear (NTE): the ear that we want to "keep busy" with the masking noise

Occlusion effect: the enhancement of bone conduction thresholds when the ears become occluded

Test ear (TE): the ear for which we want to obtain the threshold

Please refer to the glossary at the end of this book for more terms and definitions.

THE NITTY-GRITTY OF MASKING

This chapter is the down and dirty, nitty-gritty of masking and how to mask. As you may already know from studying for the written portion of your state examination, the concept of masking can be very involved, very confusing, and very difficult to apply. There are whole books dedicated to this one concept, and because of how involved the concept is, it scares most people half to death. It is the one concept in the field of hearing aid dispensing that I believe many people do not understand entirely and very few can even discuss or apply properly. Speaking from experience of teaching and coaching over the years, many people come to me not knowing how or when to perform masking. Many times they do not know why they are performing masking the way they are, as they are taught by those in the field who do not understand it themselves, and it is unfortunate because it is an extremely important part of obtaining valid test results.

If you are training and/or practicing for your state exam and are getting assistance from someone in the field, ask that person what he or she knows about masking. Why do we mask? What are the rules of masking and how much masking do we use and why? If the individual cannot answer all of these questions and provide the facts to back up the answers, then that person is probably not the right person to teach you the concept of masking. If the answer given is "because that is how I was taught" or "because that is just how I have always done it," then seek help from someone else who can answer those questions.

This chapter is in no way intensive enough to teach you everything you need to know about masking. The main purpose of this chapter is to take the information that you have been studying and already know from your studies and put it all together in a practical way to assist you in performing the task of masking correctly both for your practical state examination as well as in your daily practice.

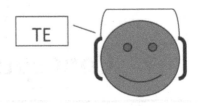

Figure 9–2. Test ear for the patient.

sound causes a wanted sound to be inaudible. When it comes to testing hearing, it is when a signal (the masking noise) is applied to the nontest ear (NTE) (Figure 9–1) in order to keep that ear from responding for the ear that is being tested (TE = test ear) (Figure 9–2). It is very important to remember that masking is required to keep a better ear busy while testing a poorer ear.

CHARACTERISTICS OF MASKING

There are things that may cause inconsistencies and roadblocks along the road of masking. The following section touches briefly on some of those variables that play a part in the masking process and terms with which you are hopefully already familiar.

Crossover occurs when you present a sound to the TE, but the NTE hears the sound first. What causes crossover? The main mechanism of crossover is presumed to be bone conduction stimulation caused by the vibration of the earphone cushion against the skull at high-stimulus intensity levels. The amount of sound that crosses over the skull is a reflection of attenuation. The interaural attenuation (IA) of air conducted tones varies depending on the frequency and earphone being used. It can differ at each frequency and varies from patient to patient. Interaural attenuation is the loss of acoustic (sound) energy of a sound as it travels from the TE across the head to the opposite ear as seen in Figure 9–3.

WHY DO WE NEED MASKING?

Although the term "masking" may be new to you, it occurs in your life on a daily basis. An example of this is you are talking to someone in your kitchen and someone turns on the dishwasher. That person is not loud enough for you to hear and understand over the noise of the dishwasher. The dishwasher (the masker) masks out the speech (the signal). Masking occurs when an unwanted

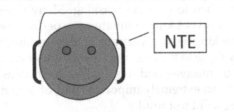

Figure 9–1. Nontest ear for the patient.

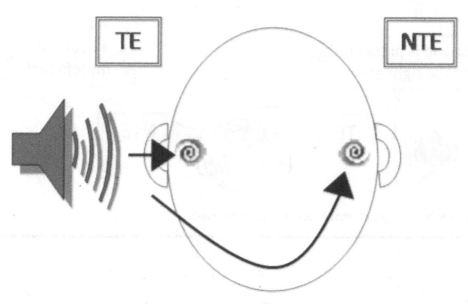

Figure 9–3. Interaural attenuation for air conduction is 40 dB HL.

- Interaural attenuation for air conduction is 40 dB HL.
- The interaural attenuation value for bone conduction is 0 dB.

So let us think about this: How loud does a 500 Hz pure tone coming out of the right earphone have to be in order for it to cross over the skull and have the left ear hear it? The left ear threshold at 500 Hz is 10 dB. The answer is 50 dB (Figure 9–4).

Overmasking is based on the IA. The easiest way to describe it would be that you have too much masking noise presented to the NTE. When this occurs, you see a shift in the threshold of the TE that would not have occurred if you had the proper amount of masking presented. Undermasking is also based on the IA. The best way to explain this characteristic is that not enough masking noise is applied to the NTE. When undermasking occurs, the NTE is responding to both the masking noise and the test signal because the masking noise is not loud enough to keep the NTE busy. In turn, this creates invalid thresholds for the TE that many times go unnoticed because the person administering the test was not knowledgeable about masking. Last but not least, we will have what is known as a masking dilemma. A masking dilemma occurs when sufficient masking from the NTE crosses over to the TE and affects threshold testing for the TE. In this case, a reliable masked threshold cannot be obtained. This generally occurs only in the presence of a substantial conductive component to the hearing loss. A masking dilemma occurs when masking is necessary but the loss makes it difficult to apply enough masking without affecting the opposite ear. This is often seen in bilateral conductive hearing losses, as seen in Figure 9–5.

What Happens If We Do Not Mask?

When testing air conduction on the poorer ear, the tone becomes loud enough to cross over the head. The good ear hears the tone.

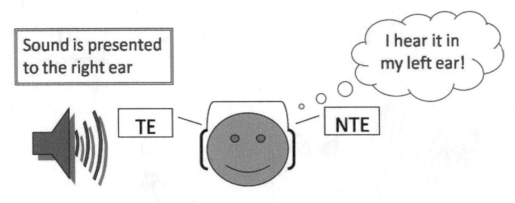

Figure 9–4. Example of what happens if we do not mask.

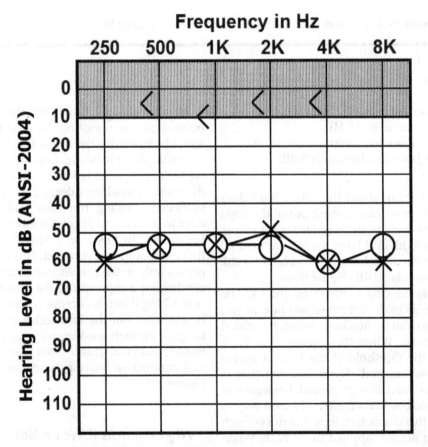

Figure 9–5. Audiogram demonstrating a masking dilemma. The intensity level required to be an effective masking level would likely create a situation resulting in overmasking. (From DeRuiter & Ramachandran, 2017)

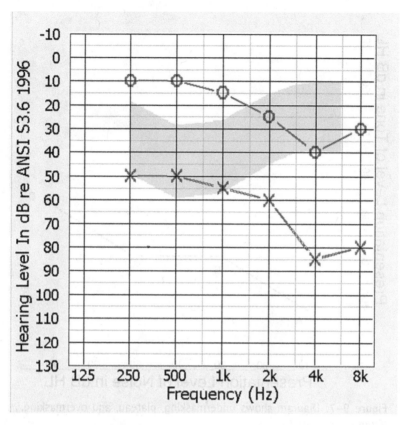

Figure 9–6. Example of a mirror audiogram is shown.

Patients may not be aware that they are hearing the tone in the good ear. They respond by raising their hand. This results in a "shadow or mirror audiogram," which is shown in Figure 9–6. The thresholds recorded are not the true thresholds of the TE. The true thresholds of the left ear are not recorded; instead, the point at which the crossover occurs is recorded. So the true threshold of the left ear cannot be established until we have masked the right ear to keep it from responding. So now let us take a look at how we go about masking to prevent this from occurring and how we go about properly masking to obtain the true thresholds.

Thresholds obtained using masking are called "masked thresholds" and should represent the true threshold of the test ear.

Effective masking (EM) eliminates crossover from occurring. Effective masking determines how much noise is appropriate to "keep the better ear busy" while you test the poorer ear (Figure 9–7.)

Undermasking occurs when the masking noise presented to the better ear is not loud enough to eliminate crossover or IA. (Undermasking occurs more commonly in air conduction testing.)

Overmasking occurs when each 10 dB increase in masking shifts the hearing threshold by 10 dB or more

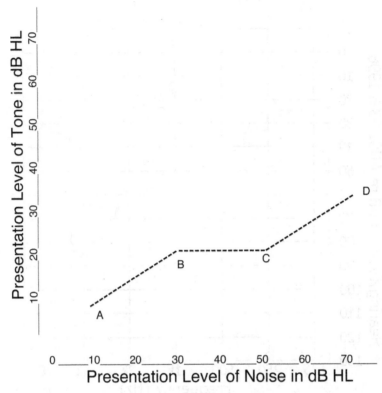

Figure 9–7. Diagram shows undermasking, plateau, and overmasking. (From Valente, 2009)

above the plateau. (Overmasking occurs more commonly in bone conduction testing.)

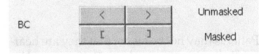

Figure 9–9. Bone conduction symbols, both unmasked and masked.

Figure 9–8 and Figure 9–9 are examples of the proper symbols that should be used to plot masked thresholds on the audiogram.

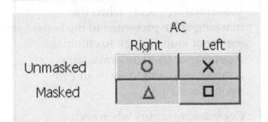

Figure 9–8. Air conduction symbols, both unmasked and masked.

RULES OF MASKING

Regarding when to mask, whenever the threshold of the poorer ear by air conduction

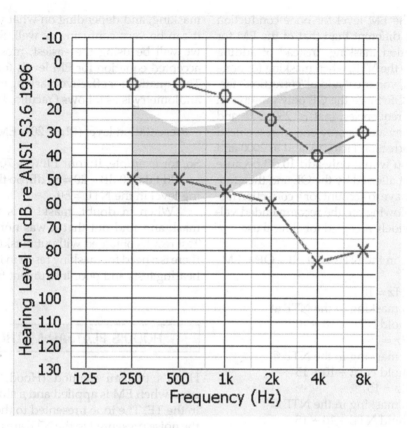

Figure 9–10. Masking is required in the better ear when the difference in air conduction thresholds between ears is 40 dB or more.

exceeds the IA of 40 dB, masking is required to obtain an accurate threshold of the poorer ear. So how much masking do we need to keep the NTE busy while presenting the signal to the TE without undermasking or overmasking when it comes to air conduction testing? The answer is 10 dB (Hood, 1960); thus, the formula for air conduction masking is:

Threshold of the NTE + 10 dB = EM level.

Rule 1: If there is a 40 dB difference in air conduction thresholds between ears, you must mask (Figure 9–10).

Anytime the NTE displays an air–bone gap, it should be masked when testing the TE. A good practice is to always mask for bone conduction.

Rule 2: Mask for bone conduction when a 15 dB or more difference occurs between the bone conduction and the air conduction.

Occlusion Effect

The occlusion effect (OE) may cause bone conduction thresholds to shift once headphones are placed on the head. Because of this phenomenon, we must account for the amount of increase we will see in the bone conduction scores by increasing the level of the masking noise. So the EM level for bone conduction masking is different than that of the EM for air conduction masking. Instead of adding the 10 dB to the NTE, when masking for bone conduction, you must add a "correction" factor for the OE. Since the OE only presents in the lower frequencies, that is, 250, 500, and 1000 Hz, they are the only ones that we need to add a correction factor to, and at 2000 and 4000 Hz you would only add 10 dB because they are not affected by the OE and therefore we do not have to account for a correction factor. The following are the recommended values most widely accepted for clinical use:

Threshold in the NTE + 10 dB + OE = EM

- 1000 Hz = 10
  Begin masking in the NTE at threshold NTE + 10 + 10
- 500 Hz = 15
  Begin masking in the NTE @ threshold NTE + 10 + 15
- 250 Hz = 15
  Begin masking in the NTE @ threshold NTE + 10 + 15

Rule 3: If you have a 40 dB or greater difference between SRTs, or if you had to mask at two or more frequencies in the speech range, you must mask for speech.

Rule 4: If you masked for SRT, then you must mask for speech discrimination.

Masking for speech audiometry can be tricky, like with air and bone conduction

---

Correction Factors

1000 Hz threshold NTE + 20 dB = EM level

500 Hz threshold NTE + 25 dB = EM level

250 Hz threshold NTE + 25 dB = EM level

---

masking, and depending on what you read, it can be very confusing as well. So, again, we will be using the easiest, most widely accepted equation for EM levels for speech. The equation for effective masking for speech audiometry is as follows (Yacullo, 1995):

Presentation level (PL) − 20 = EM level.

So, for example, if your PL was 70 dB, you would take 70 dB − 20 = 50 dB. So the masking level in the NTE = 50.

When in doubt, mask! It is better to mask and find out that it was not needed. Test results obtained without masking when there is a need for masking result in improper hearing tests and poor instrument fittings.

HOOD'S PLATEAU METHOD

Hood's plateau method (Hood, 1960) is used when EM is applied and a shift occurs in the TE. The tone presented to the TE and the noise presented to the NTE are increased by 5 dB increments until the noise can be raised or lowered 15 dB without any shift in the TE.

Examples of How to Mask

For these examples, use a blank audiogram from the back of this manual and write out the thresholds as they are established.

Example 1

Step 1: You have established 0 dB thresholds in the right ear via air conduction thresholds across all test frequencies.

Step 2: You have also established the threshold in the poorer (left ear) at 1000 Hz at 50 dB, as shown in Figure 9–11.

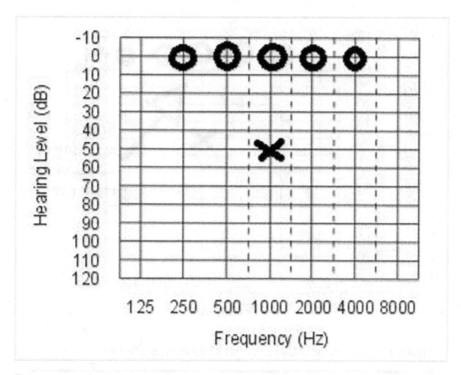

Figure 9–11. Example of 40 dB difference between air conduction thresholds.

Step 3: Determine if there is a masking rule that applies.

Step 4: If yes, which rule applies? (For this example, masking rule 1 applies because there is a 40 dB difference between air conduction thresholds.)

Step 5: What is the threshold in the NTE? (0 dB)

Step 6: How loud should we begin the masking noise in the NTE (Figure 9–12)?

- Threshold in NTE (0 dB) + 10 dB
- 0 + 10 = 10 dB will be the EM level

Step 7: Present tone to TE (50 dB). Did your patient respond?

- If yes, and the threshold does not change, then add another 5 dB of masking.

- If no, and the threshold does change, then raise the tone in the TE by 5 dB.

Step 8: Repeat step 7 until a 15 dB change in the masking level has occurred and has not shifted the tone in the TE. This threshold is then considered your true threshold for the TE.

Example 2

Step 1: You have established 35 dB thresholds in both ears via air conduction thresholds across all test frequencies.

Step 2: Testing by bone conduction, you have also established the threshold in the right ear at 1000 Hz at 10 dB.

Step 3: Determine if there is a masking rule that applies.

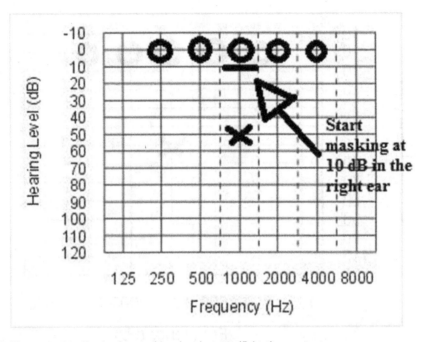

Figure 9–12. Begin the masking level at 10 dB in the nontest ear.

Step 4: If yes, which rule applies? (For this example, masking rule 2 applies because a 15 dB or more difference occurs between the bone conduction of the better ear and the air conduction of the poorer ear.)

Step 5: What is the threshold in the NTE? (35 dB in the left ear)

Step 6: How loud should we begin the masking noise in the NTE?

- Threshold in the NTE at 1000 Hz + 10 dB + OE = EM
- 35 + 10 + 10 = 55 dB
- Begin masking in the NTE at 55 dB

Step 7: Present tone to TE (10 dB). Did your patient respond?

- If yes, and the threshold does not change, then add another 5 dB of masking.

- If no, and the threshold does change, then raise the tone in the TE by 5 dB.

Step 8: Repeat step 7 until a 15 dB change in the masking level has occurred and has not shifted the tone in the TE. This threshold is then considered your true threshold for the TE.

MASKING NOISE

The last thing we need to touch on is the different types of masking noise. (Because this is just a basic overview, please review other books on masking for a more in-depth look into the differences in masking noise.) Audiometers have several kinds of masking noise to enable us to perform this task when doing an audiometric test. Types of masking noises that are generally used for testing hearing are:

1. White noise: most common; broadband noise containing equal amount of energy at all frequencies; effective for both pure tone and speech testing
2. Narrowband noise: consists of a narrow range of frequencies of equal intensity; centers around one given frequency range (i.e., testing at 250 Hz, the narrowband tones generate around 250 Hz); effective for pure-tone testing, but not effective for speech testing; the form of masking that is most widely used for pure-tone masking
3. Speech noise: white noise filtered to a low- and middle-frequency spectrum; effective for speech testing and the one that is most widely used

CONCLUSION

As discussed at the beginning of this chapter, masking is a very difficult concept to understand and apply, but it is very important to the validity of your test results. If it is not performed correctly, the results can be invalid, which would cause a misrepresentation of a hearing-loss type, degree, and configuration, as discussed in Chapters 1 and 2 (Valente, 2009).

REFERENCES

DeRuiter, M., & Ramachandran, V. (2010). *Basic audiometry learning manual* (p. 126). San Diego, CA: Plural Publishing.

Hood, J. D. (1960). The principles and practice of bone conduction audiometry. *Laryngoscope, 71*, 1211–1228.

Valente, M. (2009). *Pure-tone audiometry and masking* (p. 99). San Diego, CA: Plural Publishing.

Yacullo, W. S. (1995). *Clinical masking procedures.* Boston, MA: Allyn & Bacon.

MODULE 1

Putting It All Together

There is a hands-on audiometric section for just about every state licensing exam. Some states require a full audiometric exam performed on a test subject, whether that subject is provided by the state or required for you to bring. Other states have you perform the testing on a simulator that will respond as if a patient were sitting there with you. Review the information provided by your state so you are fully aware of what the requirements are.

Make sure that you are proficient and comfortable in performing all aspects of an audiometric examination so you are prepared for anything that the state may request of you. The time that is given for this portion of the examination varies by state, and when you are informed of that time by your state, ensure that you are able to perform the required portions in the allotted time. Practice! Practice! Practice!

Prior to taking your exam, practice performing audiometric testing on as many adults as you can. For the day of the exam, if you are required to bring a test subject, note that usually those subjects are required to be 18 years of age or older. The subjects must also present with normal hearing and their ears must be clear of debris or cerumen. Ensure that they do not exhibit any deformity or abnormality of the ear. So basically they cannot present with *any* of the FDA red flags. Make sure you are comfortable performing an otoscopic inspection of the subject's ear and that you are able to see the tympanic membrane clearly while bridging and bracing during your otoscopic examination.

As previously stated, many states require that your subject have normal hearing levels and that he or she cannot exhibit any degree of hearing loss. This is important to know because for the masking part, you *must* know the masking rules and be able to tell the proctors when you know you would need to mask because you may see normal thresholds on the exam and you will be expected to know that you need to use those thresholds when masking.

Most states will inform you of what you are required to bring to the exam and what will be provided to you. Ensure that you bring only what is asked for. For those states that require you to bring your own audiometer and tympanometer, ensure that you read the provided documentation given to you by the state prior to the exam to ensure that you are bringing *exactly* what the state requires.

EXAMPLE OF EXAM DAY WITHOUT TYMPANOMETRY

1. Wash hands before starting. Have a clean white towel next to your audiometer to place all cleaned equipment on the towel (headphones, bone oscillator, otoscope, and two clean speculum tips). Set up the equipment. Clean the headphones and bone oscillator and place them on the towel. Then take out your otoscope and two speculum tips (one for each ear), clean them, and place them on your towel. Finally, wipe down the controls (buttons, dials, etc.) of the audiometer.

   ▪ It may be best to use disposable tips that you can throw away after use.

2. Once you have your equipment set up, tell the instructor that you are going to perform a biologic check (see Chapter 6

for instructions on performing the check) of your equipment.

- When your state requires you to bring an audiometer and for you to perform a biologic check, just know that the proctors will more than likely perform a biologic check as well on your equipment.

3. After doing the biologic check, clean the headphones and bone oscillator again, and put them back on the clean white towel.

4. Invite your patient to sit down at a 90° angle away from the audiometer to perform the testing.

- Some states do not require you to bring a patient or even test on a live patient, as they use a simulator for you to perform your testing. If you are not required to bring a patient, just be aware that you will probably need to "act" like you are working with a patient, so you will be talking out loud telling the proctors what you are doing.

5. Instruct your patient that you are going to be examining her/his ear canals and then ask the eight FDA questions:

  a. State that you will be examining the outer ear for any visible deformity either congenital or traumatic.
  b. Has the patient had active drainage from the ear in the past 90 days?
  c. Has the patient experienced any acute or chronic dizziness in the past 90 days?
  d. Has the patient ever been told that she/he has a conductive hearing loss (an audiometric air–bone gap greater than or equal to 15 dB at 500, 1000, and 2000 Hz)?

  e. Has the patient ever had cerumen removed from her/his ears? (You can also let the patient know that you will be looking for any visible signs of cerumen during your otoscopic exam.)
  f. Does the patient experience a hearing loss in only one ear (unilateral hearing loss)?
  g. Has the patient experienced a sudden hearing loss in one or both ears in the past 90 days?
  h. Does the patient experience any pain or discomfort in the ears?

- These questions are just examples of the way in which you can ask your patient the FDA's eight red flag questions. Find what works best for you and stick with it; that way, the day of the exam, you are prepared.

6. Perform an otoscopic inspection of each ear and be sure to change speculum tips between ears.

7. Ask the patient if she/he has a better ear. If the patient does not know, start with the right ear.

8. Inform your patient of what you are about to do. For example: "What we are going to do is, I am going to place these headphones over your ears and you are going to hear a bunch of tones and beeps. What I want you to do is raise your hand when you hear the tones, even if they are really soft. You will first hear them in your right ear and then your left ear; as long as you hear a tone, regardless of how soft it is, raise your hand. Do you understand?"

9. Place the headphones on the patient's head, checking with two fingers for collapsed ear canals.

10. Tell the instructor what you are going to do. For example: Starting at 30 dB in the right ear at 1000 Hz, I will begin my testing; always going down 10, up 5, using

three tones at each level. I will repeat this procedure three times until I get a consistent response. This is the modified Hughson–Westlake procedure."

11. Some states may have you perform a full audiometric evaluation of your patient, whereas others may only have you perform select frequencies. Follow the instructions set forth by the state. If, for example, you are asked to only "Test both ears using air conduction at 500, 1000, and 2000 Hz," you would start with the right ear at 1000 Hz, obtain your threshold, and then test 2000 Hz, and then state that you would retest at 1000 Hz for test–retest reliability, and then proceed to test at 500 Hz. Then perform the testing on the left ear.

12. Masking air conduction: If your state requires a full audiometric exam but your air conduction thresholds do not meet the masking rule for air conduction masking, tell the proctors that you are aware of the masking rule, but for this test you will be using the thresholds that you have on your audiogram and proceed from there. Before beginning air conduction masking, sanitize your hands and remove the headphones from the patient's ears and instruct the patient on what you are going to do. If there is no patient, tell the proctors what instructions you would give to the patient if there were one present. Instructions to the patient: "What we are going to do now is, I am going to put a windy/static noise in your right/left ear (whichever one you are putting the masking in) and play the tone in the opposite ear. What I want you to do is ignore the windy noise in your right/left ear, and only raise your hand when you hear the tone in the opposite ear, even if it is really soft. Do you understand?"

13. Once completed, sanitize your hands and remove the headphones from the patient's ears and place them back on the towel.

14. Wash your hands before starting bone conduction testing. When placing the bone oscillator on the patient's head, be sure to mention that you are checking to make sure that the oscillator is not touching the pinna or hair. Place the bone oscillator on the mastoid and place the other end on the opposite temple. Instruct the patient on what you are going to do. For example: "What we are going to do now is, I am going to play some more tones and beeps for you, and again they will start off loud and get softer and softer. Raise your hand when you hear the tone, even when it is soft. This time it does not matter where you hear the tone; as long as you hear the tone, raise your hand. Do you understand?" Proceed with testing as put forth by your state.

15. If you need to or are asked by your state to perform bone conduction masking, explain to the proctors that you are using Hood's plateau method to find the test results. In the NTE (ear with masking), increase the tone up by 5 dB. When the TE threshold stays the same and you have increased the NTE by 15 dB, you have reached threshold. As with the air conduction masking, your audiogram will more than likely not meet the masking rule for bone conduction masking, and you must state to the proctors that you will be using the thresholds on your audiogram and let them know that you in fact know what the rule is for bone conduction masking and tell them what the rule is.

16. Speech reception threshold (SRT) testing. After performing pure-tone testing, determine what your pure-tone average (PTA) is and then start your testing 40 dB above your PTA. Make sure you state out loud to the proctors how you are determining your starting level for testing so that you prove to the state that you know what you are doing and why.

The following are steps for testing SRT using sanitary means for both you and your patient:

- Wash your hands.
- Remove the bone oscillator from the patient's head and place it back on your sanitary surface.
- Instruct your patient as to what you are about to do. For example: "What we are going to do now is, I am going to present a list of words to you in each ear. The words will start off loud and then get softer and softer. What I would like you to do is repeat the word back to me as best you can. It is acceptable to take a guess if you must. We will start with your right ear and then test your left ear. Do you understand?"
- Place the headphone on the patient's head.
- First determine the patient's PTA based on the pure-tone thresholds and start your SRT testing 40 dB above the PTA. (If the threshold is not known, then start at 50 dB HL.)
- Start by familiarizing the patient with the words at the starting level by presenting approximately 10 words to get she or he comfortable.
- Then, in 10 dB descending steps, present one spondee word at a time. If the patient repeats it correctly, then decrease in 10 dB steps until the patient misses a word.
- When the patient misses a word, increase the level 5 dB and present one spondee word. If the patient misses, then increase another 5 dB until a correct response.
- Once you obtain a correct response, decrease in 10 dB increments and repeat steps 7 and 8.
- When you have presented one spondee at each level and have obtained a correct response three

times, this is considered your threshold.
- Mark your SRT in the proper place on the audiogram.
- Once you have obtained your threshold in the right ear, repeat steps 5 to 11 on the left ear.

17. Speech discrimination

The following steps are for performing speech discrimination/word recognition testing:

1. Determine the level at which you are going to be presenting the word list.
2. Instruct your patient as to what you are going to be doing. For example: "What we are going to do now is, I am going to present some more words to you. This time the words will not get any softer; they are going to stay at one level. What I would like you to do is repeat the word back to me as best you can. I will be presenting the words at the end of a phrase; I will say, "Say the word__" and I would like you to only repeat the word to me at the end of the phrase as best you can, and you can take a guess if you have to, if you are unsure of the word you heard. Do you understand?"
3. Test starting with the patient's better ear, unless the hearing loss is symmetrical, then start with the right ear. Present the list of 50 words keeping track of every word that the patient repeats incorrectly.
4. After you have presented all 50 words, count the incorrect words (remember that each incorrect word is worth two points) and subtract by 100, and that is your speech discrimination score for that ear.
5. Mark your score in the appropriate area on your audiogram.
6. Repeat steps 1 to 6 on the opposite ear. (You can skip step 2, since you have already instructed the patient.)

18. Most comfortable loudness (MCL)

The following steps are for performing MCL testing:

1. Testing is done by starting 40 dB above the SRT at about the same level that you performed your speech discrimination/word recognition testing.
2. Start with the better ear first, unless the hearing loss is symmetrical, then start with the right ear.
3. Instruct the patient on what you are going to do. For example: "What we are going to do now is, I am going to continually talk to you, and what I want to find out is the level at which it is most comfortable for you to listen to me. So at the level that my voice is at right now, if I were a television and you had to listen to me, would you turn me up, turn me down, or leave me just where I am?"
4. Depending on the response you get, you will increase or decrease the level by 5 dB and ask the patient how your voice sounds and if it is at a comfortable level.
5. Once you have established the level at which the patient feels most comfortable, mark it in the appropriate place on the audiogram.
6. Repeat steps 1 to 5 on the opposite ear.

19. Testing uncomfortable loudness level (UCL). First you must turn the chair around and have the patient facing you. You are doing this so you can watch the facial cues and gestures of the patient as you are presenting the tones. Instruct the patient: "What we are going to do now is, you are going to hear some more tones and beeps. We are going to start with your right ear and then we will test your left ear. This time the tones are going to start off loud, and then they will continue to get louder and louder. What I would like you to do is raise one finger when you feel the tone is loud, and then, when you feel the tone is uncomfortably loud where you would not want to listen to it anymore, raise your whole hand, and I will stop. So, one finger for loud, whole hand for uncomfortable, do you understand?" Start at 70 dB. Present the tones in pairs of short bursts, pausing no longer than 1 second. Raise the tone in 5 dB increments until the patient raises a hand or you witness a change in the patient's expression such as wincing, head jerks, and so forth. Record the value on your audiogram according to the audiogram legend.

The following steps are for obtaining UCL by tones at each frequency:

1. When testing UCL using tones by frequency, they are generally obtained in each ear at 500, 1000, 2000, and 4000 Hz.
2. Begin by testing the better ear, unless the ears are symmetrical, then start with the right ear.
3. Instruct the patient on what you are going to do. For example: "What we are doing to do now is, I am going to present some tones to you. The tones will start off loud and continue to get louder and louder. What I would like you to do is to raise your finger when you feel that the tone is loud, and when you feel the tone is uncomfortably loud where you would not want to listen to it anymore, raise your whole hand, and I will stop. So raise your finger for loud, and raise your whole hand for uncomfortably loud, and I will stop. Do you understand?"
4. Begin at 70 dB HL or at the known level of MCL by tone at 1000 Hz, and present the tone by pulsing it in 5 dB increments until the patient responds by raising a whole hand, you have reached the limit of the audiometer, or you have visually

recognized that the patient is experiencing discomfort.

5. Once you have obtained that response, mark it on the audiogram using the symbol provided in the legend on the correct frequency for UCL.

6. You will then continue testing at 2000, 4000, and 500 Hz, recording your findings.

7. Once you have completed testing on one ear, follow steps 4 to 6 on the opposite ear.

20. When you have finished the testing, thank the patient. Clean your equipment again before placing it in your audiometer, and thank your patient once more.

EXAMPLE OF EXAM DAY WITH TYMPANOMETRY

1. Wash hands before starting. Have a clean white towel next to your audiometer and tympanometer to place all cleaned equipment on the towel (headphones, bone oscillator, otoscope, different size probe tips and two clean speculum tips). Set up the equipment. Clean the headphones and bone oscillator and place them on the towel. Then take out your otoscope and two speculum tips (one for each ear), clean them, and place them on your towel. Take out the case with the various size probe tips and open it up. Finally, wipe down the controls (buttons, dials, etc.) of the audiometer and tympanometer.

   ▪ It may be best to use disposable tips that you can throw away after use.

2. Once you have your equipment set up, tell the instructor that you are going to perform a biologic check (see Chapter 6 for instructions on performing the check) of your equipment.

   ▪ When your state requires you to bring an audiometer and for you to perform a biologic check, just know that the proctors will more than likely perform a biologic check as well on your equipment.

3. After doing the biologic check, clean the headphones and bone oscillator again, and put them back on the clean white towel.

4. Invite your patient to sit down as you face her or him at a 90° angle away from the audiometer to perform the testing.

   ▪ Some states do not require you to bring a patient or even test on a live patient, as they use a simulator for you to perform your testing. If you are not required to bring a patient, just be aware that you will probably need to "act" like you are working with a patient, so you will be talking out loud telling the proctors what you are doing.

5. Instruct your patient that you are going to be examining her/his ear canals and then ask the eight FDA questions:

   a. State that you will be examining the outer ear for any visible deformity either congenital or traumatic.

   b. Has the patient had active drainage from the ear in the past 90 days?

   c. Has the patient experienced any acute or chronic dizziness in the past 90 days?

   d. Has the patient ever been told that she/he has a conductive hearing loss (an audiometric air–bone gap greater than or equal to 15 dB at 500, 1000, and 2000 Hz)?

   e. Has the patient ever had cerumen removed from her/his ears? (You can also let the patient know that you will be looking for any visible signs of cerumen during your otoscopic exam.)

f. Has the patient experienced a hearing loss in only one ear (unilateral hearing loss)?

g. Has the patient experienced a sudden hearing loss in one or both ears in the past 90 days?

h. Does the patient experience any pain or discomfort in their ears?

- These questions are just examples of the way in which you can ask your patient the FDA's eight red flag questions. Find what works best for you and stick with it; that way, the day of the exam, you are prepared.

6. Perform an otoscopic inspection of each ear and be sure to change specula tips between ear.

7. Steps for obtaining a tympanogram:

1. Choose the appropriate size probe based on the patient ear canal size.
2. Insert probe into ear canal ensuring there is an air-tight seal.
3. Once the seal is made, a steady 226 Hz tone is presented at 85 dBSPL.
4. The air pump then adjusts the pressure equal to +200 daPa and at that time take a measurement of the compliance.
5. As the pressure is increased, the tympanic membrane and ossicular chain stiffen due to the pressure.
6. At that time, successive measurements are made of compliance as the pressure is decreased.
7. Once the pressure has reached 0 daPa or atmospheric pressure, negative pressure is created by the pump.
8. As the pressure changes occur, compliance measurements are made along the way.

8. Ask the patient if she/he have a better ear. If the patient does not know, start with the right ear.

9. Inform your patient of what you are about to do. For example: "What we are going to do is, I am going to place these headphones over your ears and you are going to hear a bunch of tones and beeps. What I want you to do is raise your hand when you hear the tones, even if they are really soft. You will first hear them in your right ear and then your left ear; as long as you hear a tone, regardless of how soft it is, raise your hand. Do you understand?"

10. Place the headphones on the patient's head, checking with two fingers for collapsed ear canals.

11. Tell the instructor what you are going to do. For example: "Starting at 30 dB in the right ear at 1000 Hz, I will begin my testing; always going down 10, up 5, using three tones at each level. I will repeat this procedure three times until I get a consistent response. This is the modified Hughson–Westlake procedure."

12. Some states may have you perform a full audiometric evaluation of your patient, whereas others may only have you perform select frequencies. Follow the instructions set forth by the state. If, for example, the proctors ask you to only "Test both ears using air conduction at 500, 1000, and 2000 Hz," you would start with the right ear at 1000 Hz, obtain your threshold, and then test 2000 Hz, and then state that you would retest at 1000 Hz for test–retest reliability, and then proceed to test at 500 Hz. Then perform the testing on the left ear.

13. Masking air conduction: If your state requires a full audiometric exam but your air conduction thresholds do not meet the masking rule for air conduction masking, tell the proctors that you are aware of the masking rule, but for this test you will be using the thresholds that you have on your audiogram and proceed from there. Before beginning air conduction masking, sanitize your hands and remove the headphones from the patient's ears and instruct the

patient on what you are going to do. If there is no patient, tell the proctors what instructions you would give to the patient if there were one present. Instructions to the patient: "What we are going to do now is, I am going to put a windy/static noise in your right/ left ear (whichever one you are putting the masking in) and play the tone in the opposite ear. What I want you to do is ignore the windy noise in your right/left ear, and only raise your hand when you hear the tone in the opposite ear, even if it is really soft. Do you understand?"

14. Once completed, sanitize your hands and remove the headphones from the patient's ears and place them back on the towel.

15. Wash your hands before starting bone conduction testing. When placing the bone oscillator on the patient's head, be sure to mention that you are checking to make sure that the oscillator is not touching the pinna or hair. Place the bone oscillator on the mastoid and place the other end on the opposite temple. Instruct the patient on what you are going to do. For example: "What we are going to do now is, I am going to play some more tones and beeps for you, and again they will start off loud and get softer and softer. Raise your hand when you hear the tone, even when it is soft. This time it does not matter where you hear the tone; as long as you hear the tone, raise your hand. Do you understand?" Proceed with testing as put forth by your state.

16. If you need to or are asked by your state to perform bone conduction masking, explain to the proctors that you are using Hood's plateau method to find the test results. In the NTE (ear with masking) increase the tone up by 5 dB. When the TE threshold stays the same and you have increased the NTE by 15 dB, you have reached threshold. As with the air conduction masking, your audiogram will more than likely not meet the masking rule for bone conduction masking, and you must state to the proctors that you will be using the thresholds on your audiogram and let them know that you in fact know what the rule is for bone conduction masking and tell them what the rule is.

17. Speech reception threshold (SRT) testing. After performing pure-tone testing, determine what your pure-tone average (PTA) is and then start your testing 40 dB above your PTA. Make sure you state out loud to the proctors how you are determining your starting level for testing so that you prove to the state that you know what you are doing and why.

The following are steps for testing SRT using sanitary means for both you and your patient:

1. Wash your hands.
2. Remove the bone oscillator from the patient's head and place it back on your sanitary surface.
3. Instruct your patient as to what you are about to do. For example: "What we are going to do now is, I am going to present a list of words to you in each ear. The words will start off loud and then get softer and softer. What I would like you to do is repeat the word back to me as best you can. It is acceptable to take a guess if you must. We will start with your right ear and then test your left ear. Do you understand?"
4. Place the headphone on the patient's head.
5. First determine the patient's PTA based on the pure-tone thresholds and start your SRT testing 40 dB above the PTA. (If the threshold is not known, then start at 50 dB HL.)
6. Start by familiarizing the patient with the words at the starting level by presenting approximately 10 words to get the patient comfortable.

7. Then, in 10 dB descending steps, present one spondee word at a time. If the patient repeats it correctly, then decrease in 10 dB steps until the patient misses a word.

8. When the patient misses a word, increase the level 5 dB and present one spondee word. If the patient misses, then increase another 5 dB until a correct response.

9. Once you obtain a correct response, decrease in 10 dB increments and repeat steps 7 and 8.

10. When you have presented one spondee at each level and have obtained a correct response three times, this is considered your threshold.

11. Mark your SRT in the proper place on the audiogram.

12. Once you have obtained your threshold in the right ear, repeat steps 5 to 10 on the left ear.

18. Speech discrimination

The following steps are for performing speech discrimination/word recognition testing:

1. Determine the level at which you are going to be presenting the word list.

2. Instruct your patient as to what you are going to be doing. For example: "What we are going to do now is, I am going to say some more words to you. This time the words will not get any softer; they are going to stay at one level. What I would like you to do is repeat the word back to me as best you can. I will be presenting the words at the end of a phrase; I will say, "Say the word_____" and I would like you to only repeat the word to me at the end of the phrase as best you can, and you can take a guess if you have to, if you are unsure of the word you heard. Do you understand?"

3. Test starting with the patient's better ear, unless the hearing loss is symmetrical, then start with the right ear. Present the list of 50 words keeping track of every word that the patient repeats incorrectly.

4. After you have presented all 50 words, count the incorrect words (remember that each incorrect word is worth two points) and subtract by 100, and that is your speech discrimination score for that ear.

5. Mark your score in the appropriate area on your audiogram.

6. Repeat steps 1 to 6 on the opposite ear. (You can skip step 2, since you have already instructed the patient.)

19. Most comfortable loudness (MCL)

The following steps are for performing MCL testing:

1. Testing is done by starting 40 dB above the SRT at about the same level that you performed your speech discrimination/word recognition testing.

2. Start with the better ear first, unless the hearing loss is symmetrical, then start with the right ear.

3. Instruct the patient on what you are going to do. For example: "What we are going to do now is, I am going to continually talk to you, and what I want to find out is the level at which it is most comfortable for you to listen to me. So at the level that my voice is at right now, if I were a television and you had to listen to me, would you turn me up, turn me down, or leave me just where I am?"

4. Depending on the response that you get, you will increase or decrease the level by 5 dB and ask the patient how your voice sounds and if it is at a comfortable level.

5. Once you have established the level at which the patient feels most comfortable, mark it in the appropriate place on the audiogram.

6. Repeat steps 1 to 5 on the opposite ear.

20. Testing uncomfortable loudness level (UCL). First you must turn the chair around and have the patient facing you. You are doing this so you can watch the facial cues and gestures of the patient as you are presenting the tones. Instruct the patient: "What we are going to do now is, you are going to hear some more tones and beeps. We are going to start with your right ear and then we will test your left ear. This time the tones are going to start off loud, and then they will continue to get louder and louder. What I would like you to do is raise one finger when you feel the tone is loud, and then, when you feel the tone is uncomfortably loud where you would not want to listen to it anymore, raise your whole hand, and I will stop. So, one finger for loud, whole hand for uncomfortable, do you understand?" Start at 70 dB. Present the tones in pairs of short bursts, pausing no longer than 1 second. Raise the tone in 5 dB increments until the patient raises a hand or you witness a change in the patient's expression such as wincing, head jerks, and so forth. Record the value on your audiogram according to the audiogram legend.

The following steps are for obtaining UCL by tones at each frequency:

1. When testing UCL using tones by frequency, they are generally obtained in each ear at 500, 1000, 2000, and 4000 Hz.
2. Begin by testing the better ear, unless the ears are symmetrical, then start with the right ear.
3. Instruct the patient on what you are going to do. For example: "What we are doing to do now is, I am going to present some tones to you. The tones will start off loud and continue to get louder and louder. What I would like you to do is to raise

your finger when you feel that the tone is loud, and when you feel the tone is uncomfortably loud where you would not want to listen to it anymore, raise your whole hand, and I will stop. So raise your finger for loud, and raise your whole hand for uncomfortably loud, and I will stop. Do you understand?"

4. Begin at 70 dB HL or at the known level of MCL by tone at 1000 Hz, and present the tone by pulsing it in 5 dB increments until the patient responds by raising a whole hand, you have reached the limit of the audiometer, or you have visually recognized that the patient is experiencing discomfort.
5. Once you have obtained that response, mark it on the audiogram using the symbol provided in the legend on the correct frequency for UCL.
6. You will then continue testing at 2000, 4000, and 500 Hz recording your findings.
7. Once you have completed testing on one ear, follow steps 4 to 6 on the opposite ear.

21. When you have finished the testing, thank the patient. Clean your equipment again before placing it in your audiometer, and thank your patient once more.

*A note about MCL and UCL testing: What is provided here is just an example of performing testing. It is your responsibility to READ ALL the information provided to you from your state prior to practicing for the test. Many states will provide you with exactly what they want you to do and how they want you to do it. This may include giving you the instructions on how to instruct your patient.

Congratulations, you have now completed the audiometric section of your state exam!

MODULE 1 TEST QUESTIONS

1. Which of the following is true about a mixed hearing loss?
   a. Bone scores are poorer than air scores
   b. Air and bone are both below normal, but there is an ABG
   c. Air and bone are both below normal and essentially the same
   d. None of the above

2. A sensorineural hearing loss is due to a disorder in the:
   a. Middle ear
   b. Outer ear
   c. Inner ear
   d. Eustachian tube

3. Cleaning is:
   a. Killing germs 100% of the time
   b. Killing germs 50% of the time
   c. Preparation for disinfecting and may not kill germs at all
   d. All of the above

4. Which is a common configuration for someone that has been exposed to noise?
   a. Corner audiogram
   b. Ski-slope
   c. Reverse slope
   d. Noise notch

5. An asymmetrical hearing loss is:
   a. When the characteristics of degree and configuration of the loss are different in both ears
   b. When there is a loss of hearing in only 1 ear
   c. When the hearing loss changes over time
   d. When the hearing loss presents slowly over time

6. An air–bone gap always presents with better hearing by air conduction then bone conduction.
   a. True
   b. False

7. The different characteristics of hearing loss are:
   a. Type, degree, and configuration
   b. Conductive, mixed, and sensorineural
   c. Flat, corner, and ski-slope
   d. All of the above

8. Hearing loss only occurs when both air and bone scores are below normal.
   a. True
   b. False

9. There are three possible routes for sound to travel to the ear.
   a. True
   b. False

10. What are the types of hearing loss?
    a. Mild, moderate, and severe
    b. Noise notch, flat, and precipitous
    c. Masked and unmasked
    d. Conductive, mixed, and sensorineural

11. Bone conduction is:
    a. When sound travels to the inner ear by using headphones
    b. When sound travels to the inner ear by way of the mastoid bone
    c. When sound travels to the inner ear by way of the outer and middle ear
    d. All of the above

12. The correct symbol for masked bone conduction for the left ear is:
    a. <
    b. >
    c. {
    d. }

13. When you do not get a response from a patient, you should not mark anything on the audiogram.
    a. True
    b. False

14. Threshold is:
    a. The first tone that the patient responds to
    b. The last tone that the patient responds to

c. The softest level that the patient can hear 100% of the time

d. The softest level that the patient can hear 50% of the time

15. Only a black color pen should be used to mark your symbols on the audiogram.
    a. True
    b. False

16. Although some symbols are universal, you should always read the information provided by your state to see if they recommended something different.
    a. True
    b. False

17. Which of the following is NOT an FDA red flag?
    a. Dizziness
    b. Pain in the ear
    c. Tinnitus
    d. Hearing loss in one ear

18. Which of the following is NOT a disorder of the outer ear?
    a. Dermatitis
    b. Otosclerosis
    c. Exostoses
    d. Polyps

19. It's not important to know the FDA red flags for my state exam.
    a. True
    b. False

20. Why is it important to know the FDA red flags?
    a. To know how to diagnosis a disorder
    b. To know what kind of hearing aid to recommend
    c. To know when to refer or not to refer
    d. It's not important

21. It is NOT important to refer others if they have a foreign object in the ear. You should just remove it and continue with your patient.
    a. True
    b. False

22. You should visually inspect the outer ear and mastoid process during an otoscopic exam.
    a. True
    b. False

23. When performing an otoscopic inspection, you should always:
    a. Ensure that all of your equipment is place on a sterile towel or surface
    b. Wash hands thoroughly before contact with the patient
    c. Only use one specula tip per ear
    d. All of the above

24. The technique that is used for safely holding equipment being used on a patient is called:
    a. FDA technique
    b. Otoscopic technique
    c. Bridge-and-brace technique
    d. Brace-the-head technique

25. You should perform a biologic check of your equipment:
    a. Every year
    b. Once a month
    c. Once a week
    d. Every day

26. Why is a biologic check of your equipment important?
    a. It's not important
    b. To ensure that the equipment is functioning properly
    c. To make sure it will turn on
    d. To make sure the lights turn on

27. Tympanometry:
    a. Identifies the hearing acuity of the patient
    b. Measures the static compliance of the eustachian tube
    c. Measures the dynamic compliance of the TM
    d. Measures the central processing of the middle ear.

28. Type-B tympanogram can indicate:
    a. Otitis media
    b. Cerumen impaction/occlusion
    c. The presence of a patent pressure equalization tube
    d. A perforation of the tympanic membrane
    e. All the above

29. Tympanometry is effective in identifying:
    a. Middle ear pathologies
    b. Cochlear pathologies
    c. VIIIth cranial nerve pathologies
    d. All the above

30. Which of the following is NOT true when it comes to hand washing?
    a. Wash hands only after each patient
    b. Wash hands before and after situations when you are handling hearing aids, impressions, earmolds, etc.
    c. Wash hands before and after removing and handling ear impressions
    d. Wash hands immediately after the removal of glove
    e. All of the above

For more quiz questions for Module 1, visit the companion website and test your knowledge.

MODULE 2

Ear Impressions

10

Otoscopic Inspection for Impression

Objectives

- To prepare the candidate to be knowledgeable about the purpose of performing an otoscopic inspection
- To prepare the candidate to be knowledgeable about the proper procedures used for performing an otoscopic inspection
- To prepare the candidate to be able to identify conditions suitable for ear impressions
- To ensure that the candidate is taking hygienic precautions

OTOSCOPY

As discussed in detail in Chapter 5, the first step in your otoscopic examination of the patient should always be a thorough inspection of the outer ear, which includes behind the ear. The reason for this is that the condition of the outer ear is of the utmost importance when considering the results of your audiometric test, in determining when to refer or not to refer the patient for a medical evaluation, in selecting the appropriate amplification for the patient, and lastly, for impression taking. If it has been a while since you have read and reviewed Chapter 5, I recommend that you do it at this time before continuing to read this chapter.

The main purpose of performing the otoscopic examination prior to taking an ear impression is to learn some important information about the patient's ear, such as:

- The shape of the ear and the ear canal, and how it bends and contours
- The texture of the skin and whether it is thin or not
- The diameter and length of the canal and what direction the bends may take
- Whether or not there are any issues or problems with the ear that would prevent you from taking the impression
- What size and type of otoblock you will be using

Inspection of the Outer Ear

Before inserting the otoscope tip into the ear canal, the outer ear is inspected, including behind the pinna, for any signs of malformation or anything else that would prevent you from taking an ear impression. For example, if the complaint of ear pain exists, there may be evidence of an infection of the outer ear in the form of redness or slight swelling. (See Figure 10–1 for landmarks of the outer ear.)

Examination of the External Auditory Canal

The examination is performed by using the proper bridge-and-brace technique for patient safety. The normal external auditory canal has some hair, often lined with yellow to brown wax. The total length of the ear canal in adults is approximately 1 inch (2.5 cm) and ends at the tympanic membrane (Taylor

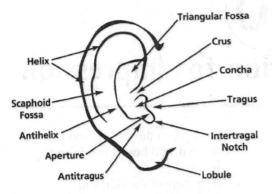

Figure 10–1. Landmarks of the outer ear are shown. (From Taylor & Mueller, 2011)

& Mueller, 2011). The first third of the ear canal is cartilage and the other two-thirds is bony and covered with a thin layer of skin.

When performing your inspection, remember the disorders of the ear that were discussed in Chapter 3, as these are conditions that you will be looking for throughout your otoscopic examination. Other conditions to consider are excessive growth of hair in the ear canal, enlarged ear canal cavity,

prolapsed ear canal, and aural discharge and inflammation of the outer ear and/or ear canal. As mentioned in Chapter 5, but important enough to mention again, make sure that the subject you bring to the exam has healthy, normal ears with no obstruction.

Examination of the Eardrum

When performing an otoscopic examination and viewing the tympanic membrane through an otoscope, the normal eardrum appears pinkish-gray in color and is circular in shape. The first of the three small bones (malleus) that transmit sound vibrations to the cochlea lies against the far side of the eardrum and can be seen through it in the upper part, like clock hands at approximately the 12 o'clock position (Figure 10–2).

Other abnormal findings seen with the otoscope include:

1. A hole (perforation) in the eardrum (depending on the cause, eardrum perforations can heal remarkably well)

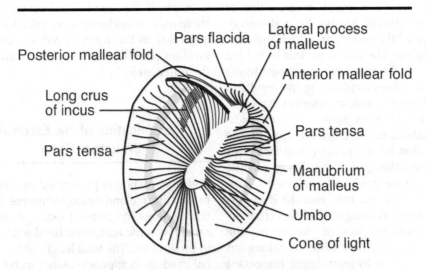

Figure 10–2. Drawing of a tympanic membrane. (From Pasha, 2011)

2. Acute infection of the middle ear (acute otitis media), which will cause the eardrum to appear abnormal in color
3. Eardrum retraction, which causes the eardrum to appear as if it is sucked in and wrapped around the malleus
4. Eardrum distention, which is caused by swelling or ballooning of the eardrum due to a buildup of fluid in the middle ear

The appearance of the eardrum in acute otitis media is dependent on the length of time that the infection has been present. Typically, the eardrum becomes red or yellow in appearance and is opaque with indistinct landmarks; it can appear to be bulging toward the viewer. Insufflation may show decreased mobility.

Sometimes in acute otitis media the eardrum will burst, allowing the pressure (and the pain) to reduce. Then one can often see the tear in the drum, as well as the discharge in the outer ear. In the majority of people, such a tear heals completely. If you have a patient who presents with any of these conditions, medical referral and medical clearance should be obtained before taking an ear impression.

Once you have performed the otoscopic inspection and have determined that the patient's ears are healthy and free from anything that would otherwise prevent you from performing the impressions, you are ready to proceed with the impressions.

REFERENCES

Pasha, R. (2011). *Otolaryngology head and neck surgery: Clinical reference guide* (3rd ed., p. 338). San Diego, CA: Plural Publishing.

Taylor, B., & Mueller, H. G. (2011). *Fitting and dispensing hearing aids*. San Diego, CA: Plural Publishing, Inc.

(11)

Ear Impression Preparation

Objectives

- To ensure that the candidate is taking hygienic precautions during the ear impression process
- To ensure that the candidate is aware of, and is following, all safety precautions during the ear impression process
- To prepare the candidate to produce a complete and accurate ear impression

OTOSCOPIC EXAMINATION PROCEDURE

One of the most important skills to acquire in order to become a competent hearing aid dispenser is taking good-quality ear impressions. There are two main reasons for becoming comfortable and competent in this area:

1. It determines the fit of the custom earmold or hearing aid that you will be fitting on the patient. It determines the experience that your patient has with the first fit and could be the factor in the patient's acceptance of amplification, so you should do everything in your power to get the impression done right the first time the patient is in your office. Remember, you are the professional, and if you take an impression and it is not good, do not be afraid to take another impression. Do not send poor impressions to the manufacturers and expect that they can fix your poor impression, because

they cannot, nor is it their responsibility to do so, it is yours!

2. Taking an ear impression is the most invasive procedure that you will be performing on your patient as a hearing aid dispenser, so precision and accuracy during the process is of the utmost importance when it comes to patient safety. There is a risk of physical harm to the patient if this procedure is not done properly, so states will be very particular when it comes to this section on the exam, as the patient's safety is the number one priority.

EQUIPMENT CHECKLIST

Most states will provide you with an equipment checklist that you are required to bring to your examination. They will also include a list of what they provide as well. Below is a list of what most states require you to bring to the examination. This equipment includes but is not limited to:

- Otoscope
- Specula tips (at least 10)
- Sanitary wipes
- Hand sanitizer
- Impression material (enough for two impressions)
- Impression mixing tools
- Syringes (2) or impression gun
- Syringe tips (2) or mixing tips for gun (4)
- Otoblocks of various sizes
- Otolight
- Sanitary cloth (white towel)
- Scissors
- Order form
- Manufacturer shipping box

The first thing you need to determine prior to taking an ear impression is what type of impression material you are going to be using when you take your state licensing examination. Do not assume that the impression material that you have been using and practicing with is approved under materials that the state allows. Consult the information on the impression-taking section of your state information prior to the exam date so that if you need to change the impression material you are using, you have plenty of time to work with a different type in advance. The main issue that states have with certain impression material is not the actual material that is used but the way in which the material is mixed and/or injected into the ear.

There are two main types of materials for taking ear impressions. The first one is a silicone-based material that can come in either individual packages for individual use or in bulk. The silicone material requires two equal parts: one consisting of silicone, and another that is a mixing agent that begins to harden once these two parts are mixed together. The main concern with this material is that it can be difficult to mix in a cup or bowl and usually requires that you do it by hand and then insert the material into the syringe. The problem with this method is that it requires you to abide by the utmost sanitary precautions when mixed by hand for the practical examination, and at times gloves may be required. If you do prefer to use silicone, research different types and find one that is available that may offer an alternative to hand mixing.

The other option for mixing silicone material is by using an impression gun. With the impression gun, the impression material comes in a two-part cartridge and mixes together as you "shoot" the gun. Guns can be either manually operated or come equipped with battery operation to assist with speed control. Some guns are strictly manual and require pressure and speed made only by your hand, whereas others are battery operated and can assist with speed and pressure control. Figure 11–1 shows an impression

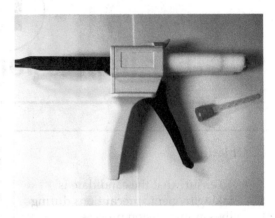

Figure 11–1. An example of an impression gun. (Courtesy of Suzanne Krumenacker)

gun. Be sure to check your state information packet before using an impression gun on your state exam, as many states do not allow impression guns during testing. (*Note.* If your state allows you to use an impression gun, make sure that you are able to properly bridge and brace while operating the gun.)

The second type of material is a powder-and-liquid material that comes either individually premeasured and prepackaged or in bulk. Mixing of the powder-and-liquid material is done using a cup or bowl. After proper mixing of the material, it is transferred to the syringe for injection. Figure 11–2 shows such a syringe. Many people find this material very easy to work with for their state exam, due to the ease of mixing and its not hardening as fast as silicone, allowing you more time to work with this material. Generally, this material does not need to be handled with your hands, as it can be transferred directly from the container after mixing into the syringe, which makes it sanitary to use without concern. (*Note.* Regardless of which material you decide to use for your exam, make sure that you read the manufacturer's instructions for the proper mixing procedure as well as setup time of the material. And don't forget to check the expiration date!!!!)

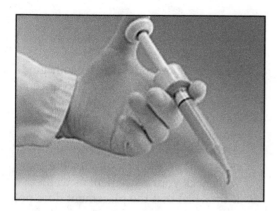

Figure 11–2. An example of a standard syringe used to take ear impressions. (From Taylor & Mueller, 2011)

Preparation Tips Prior to the Examination

1. Organize your impression kit.
2. Bring a clean white towel.
3. Place tools in separate clear bags.
4. While unpacking your tools, lay them out in order of use.
5. Sanitize every time you have to touch the patient.
6. Treat your subject as a real patient (i.e., talk to her/him during the procedure).
7. Time yourself.
8. Quality control your steps before, during, and after the procedure.

EAR IMPRESSION PROCEDURE AND STEPS

Hygiene Technique

The following points regard hygiene:

- It is very important to demonstrate the technique.
- Wash your hands before and after the procedure.
- If using gloves, be sure to wash your hands before and after use.
- It is suggested to place all items on a clean white towel (sterile surface).
- Sanitize tools and equipment prior to placing them on the sterile surface.

Explanation of the Procedure

In terms of explaining the procedure, involve the patient and explain while doing the procedure. For example: "We are now going to take an ear impression of your ear. I will be inspecting your outer ear and ear canal with my otoscope. I will be looking for any abnormalities that may stop me from performing this procedure. If all is fine, I will be placing a cotton block inside your ear canal and will then fill your ear cavity with impression material. The material will stay in your ear cavity approximately 12 minutes. Do you have any questions?"

The FDA's Eight Red Flag Questions

It is important to question the patient with regard to the following FDA red flag issues:

1. Visible congenital or traumatic deformity of the ear
2. History of active drainage from the ear in the previous 90 days
3. History of sudden or rapidly progressive hearing loss within the previous 90 days
4. Acute or chronic dizziness
5. Unilateral hearing loss of sudden or recent onset within the previous 90 days
6. Audiometric air–bone gap 5 dB at 500, 1000, and 2000 Hz
7. Visible evidence of significant cerumen accumulation or a foreign body in the ear canal
8. Pain or discomfort in the ear

Process for Otoscopic Inspection

The process for otoscopic inspection is as follows:

1. Inspect the ear canal. Use the proper bridge-and-brace technique as discussed in Chapter 5.
2. Demonstrate a clean and safe procedure for inspecting the ear structures.
3. Make sure to clean your otoscope speculum prior to touching to patient's ear.
4. Describe the entire outer ear.
5. Look for foreign objects, excessive wax, abnormal growths, and so forth, that would prevent you from taking the impression.
6. Describe the ear canal and the tympanic membrane.

Tips for During the Examination

Observe the following points during the examination:

- Talk out loud.
- Inspect each ear. Use a different speculum for each ear and sanitize it prior to placing it in the patient's ear.
- Compare what is normal for this patient's ear canals.
- Your dialog can go something like this: "I see the canal walls, which are clear and free of wax. I can see the first bend and the second bend of the canal. I can see the eardrum and the cone of light reflecting back from the light source."

Insertion of Otoblock

To insert the otoblock, do the following:

1. Select the correct-size otoblock.
2. Always bridge and brace when in contact with the patient.

3. Sanitize the otolight.
4. Gently place a cotton block in the bowl portion of the ear (Figure 11–3).
5. While bridging and bracing, gently guide the otoblock into the patient's ear canal using your otolight (Figure 11–4).
6. Reinspect block placement with the otoscope.
7. After insertion of the otoblock and your reinspection, the proctors for the exam will check your placement as well.
8. If they feel that the placement does not meet quality and safety standards for a proper and safe impression, they will

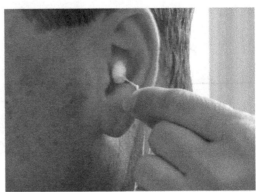

A

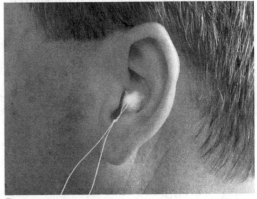

B

Figure 11–3. A. Placement of the otoblock in the bowl portion of the ear while holding the string is shown. **B.** Otoblock should be able to stay in the ear without touching it, as shown.

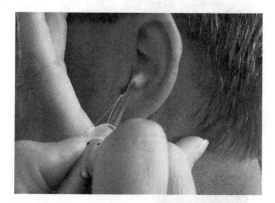

Figure 11–4. Example of bridging and bracing while using the otolight to place the block.

stop you and not allow you to actually take the impression.

Quality Assurance of Otoblock Placement

To ensure that the otoblock has been placed correctly, do the following:

- Make sure there are no gaps around the otoblock.
- Make sure that the block is firmly in place.
- Determine if the placement will yield a safe fill.
- Place the block deeply into the ear canal (must completely block eardrum).
- Do not place the block on the eardrum.
- The block should be a quarter-inch beyond the second bend, just into the bony portion of the canal.
- Placement should yield sufficient canal length.

Ear Impression Preparation

Ear impression preparation should proceed as follows:

1. Mix the impression material and place it inside of the syringe. Use a clean technique here.
2. Wash your hands with a hand sanitizer or use an antibacterial wipe if you have the putty-to-putty mixture.
3. Use a mixing bowl and spatula if using powder/liquid.
4. Transfer the material into the syringe. Ensure that there are no aid bubbles once you push the material to the end of the syringe.

When you are ready to perform the procedure, an example explanation for the patient is as follows: "You will soon feel a cool flow in your ear canal as I begin to fill your ear canal with the impression material." Make sure you describe out loud what you are doing (describe landmarks of canal, concha bowl, helix, and tragus area) as you fill the ear.

Ear Impression Procedure

The ear impression procedure is as follows:

1. Insert the syringe or gun tip inside the ear canal and begin to inject material slowly and evenly into the canal area up to the otoblock using the proper bridge-and-brace technique (Figure 11–5).
2. Once you see the material start to come back out toward the tip of the syringe, start to fill the intertragal notch, then the bowl, then the helix area, then down the tragus area, always keeping the tip of the syringe embedded into the material to avoid air bubbles or voids.
3. Continue the circular fill until the entire ear is filled.
4. Do not touch or smooth the impression with your hands. This will cause the impression to distort.
5. Let the material set for 12 minutes (or the time stated by the manufacturer of the material).
6. Look at your watch or clock to keep track of time or use a timer if one is provided.

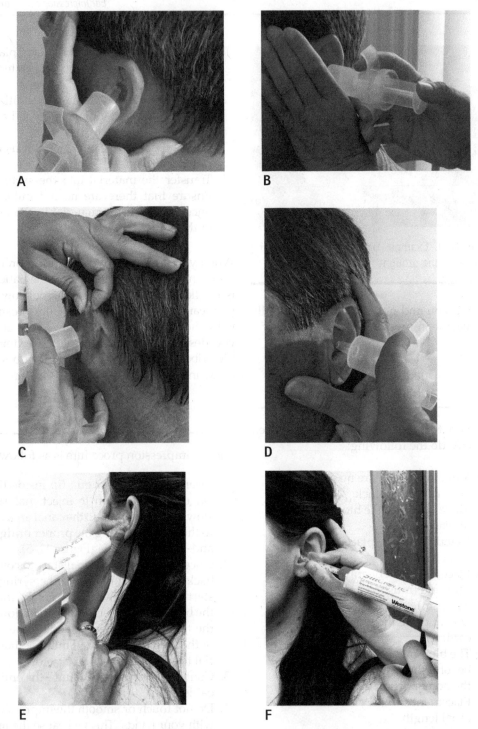

Figure 11–5. A. Example view of bridging and bracing while shooting an ear impression with syringe right handed. **B.** Different view of bridging and bracing while shooting an ear impression right handed. **C.** Example view of bridging and bracing while shooting an ear impression with syringe left handed. **D.** Different view of bridging and bracing while shooting an ear impression left handed. **E.** Example view of bridging and bracing while shooting an ear impression with gun right handed. **F.** Example view of bridging and bracing while shooting an ear impression with gun left handed.

Tips for Syringing Ear Canal

Tips for syringing the ear canal are as follows:

- Insert the syringe tip deeply without occluding the ear canal with the tip.
- Positively fill the entire canal.
- Completely fill all ear structures.
- Completely fill the outer ear.
- Completely cover the tragus lobe.
- Allow curing of the ear impression.
- Follow the manufacturer cure times.

Curing of Ear Impression

While the ear impression is curing, do the following:

1. Reclean the equipment used (otoscope, ear light, and syringe).
2. Put the syringe inside the plastic bag.
3. Wash your hands prior to removing the ear impression.

Removing the Ear Impression

To remove the ear impression, do the following:

1. Break the seal by pulling up and back on the pinna.

2. Pull the impression out of the helix area.
3. Gently lift the bottom part of the impression out of the ear so as not to stretch the earmold.
4. Pull the impression out while turning the impression toward the patient's nose.
5. The otoblock should be attached to the end of the impression upon removal. If it did not come out while removing the impression, use the string attached to the block and gently remove it from the patient's ear prior to your otoscopic inspection.

Once you have removed the ear impression from the patient's ear, clean your otoscope and reexamine the ear before doing anything else. After your inspection of the patient's ear, the proctors will inspect the ear as well to make sure the otoblock and all material have been removed and that there was no trauma inflicted on the patient during this process. For more information on impression taking, visit the companion website.

The next chapter reviews what to do once you have removed the impression from the patient's ear.

REFERENCE

Taylor, B., & Mueller, H. G. (2011). *Fitting and dispensing hearing aids* (p. 185). San Diego, CA: Plural Publishing.

12

After the Impression

Objectives

- To ensure that the candidate can determine if she/he has a good or poor impression
- To ensure that the candidate can prepare the impression to ship to a manufacturer

EVALUATING YOUR IMPRESSION

Once you have removed the ear impression from the patient's ear and have reinspected the patient's ear with your otoscope, it is time to inspect and evaluate the impression to determine if you have a good impression that can be sent to the manufacturer. I cannot stress enough here the importance of knowing the difference between a good impression and a poor impression. Experts in the industry state that some 20% of all ear impressions sent to manufacturers are poor impressions (Taylor & Mueller, 2011).

Now let us take a look at your ear impression and determine if it is of good quality. The following is a list of questions that you must ask yourself after every ear impression and especially for the day of your state examination. Figure 12–1 is a visual representation of a good impression versus poor impressions.

- Are the canal, concha, and helix filled in completely?
- Is the canal area filled completely to the otoblock, and is the otoblock attached to the end of the impression?
- Is the impression smooth and complete?
- Is the canal depth sufficient for the type of hearing aid or earmold that you are ordering?
- Can you see the beginning of the second bend?

All of these questions should be asked, but there are a couple of other things that must be looked at as well. You want to make sure that your material was properly mixed and that you do not see air bubbles on the body of the impression, and you must also check that there is a consistent color of the impression. If the material is not mixed properly, you will get colored streak marks where the material was not mixed completely or it may be overly oily depending on the material that was used.

Canal length is also extremely important to look at as well as the diameter of the canal. For an impression to be considered good, it is suggested that the canal length be beyond the second bend if at all possible. Some people consider the hearing loss that they are going to be fitting to determine how deep they are going to shoot the impression. Be very careful with this method of thinking because with a mild hearing loss, you can get by with a shorter canal that goes to the first bend, but if you are fitting a mild loss with a completely-in-the-canal (CIC) hearing aid and length is needed for retention purposes, then a short canal will not be acceptable. So the general rule of thumb is to *always* take a good long impression past the second bend and ensure that you have a complete mold of the pinna to determine if the aid will sit with all the landmarks of the pinna.

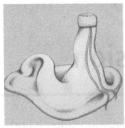

CORRECT
Canal, concha, and helix adequately filled. Canal block left attached.

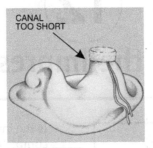

INCORRECT
Insufficient canal depth. Canal block not placed deeply enough in the ear.

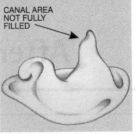

INCORRECT
Canal area not fully filled to canal block, or no block used.

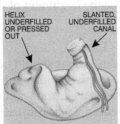

INCORRECT
Slanted underfilled canal due to improper placing of block in ear. Helix either underfilled or pressed out.

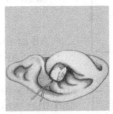

INCORRECT
Distorted due to insufficient curing time for impression, or too much liquid added to Audalin®.

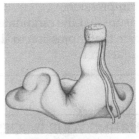

INCORRECT
Concha missing

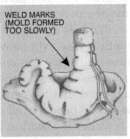

INCORRECT
Gaps or weld marks. Overall surface of impression not smooth.

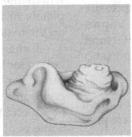

INCORRECT
Mashed or bent due to improper handling or packaging. (Not usually a problem with the silicone-based materials unless the curing time was too short.)

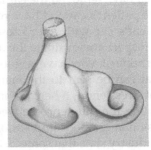

INCORRECT
Underfilled tragus

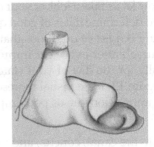

INCORRECT
Helix missing

Figure 12–1. Examples of correct versus incorrect impressions. (From Mynders, 2006)

PACKING AND SHIPPING IMPRESSION

After you have determined that the impression is of good quality and ready to send to the manufacturer, there are a few things that you need to consider. There are currently two ways that impressions can be sent to the manufacturer. One way is in an impression box, which is generally provided to you by the manufacturer, and the second way is by electronically scanning them with special equipment and e-mailing the scan to the manufacturer. Most state exams will have an impression box present as part of the materials supplied on the day of your exam and that should be "used" to ship the impression. The impression box provided by the state is generally just a prop and not for you to actually use to pack your impression. You need to tell the proctors how you would pack the impression, but you may not actually have to "do" anything.

So let us discuss what you need to know when it comes to shipping the impression using the impression box through the mail or priority shipment such as FedEx.

1. If you are using the powder-and-liquid material, know that this material is highly susceptible to temperature and can distort and even shrink if the impressions sit too long and are not shipped right away. The impressions can also be easily damaged in the shipping process if they are not packaged appropriately. If using silicone impression material, this type of material is much more durable and you do not need to be concerned with standard shipping and handling. So because of this reason, you can skip point 2.

2. Remove the inside liner from the impression box and place cement or glue on the inside liner and then adhere the impression to the glue with the impression facing straight up in the middle of the liner. If the impression has a thin canal, put a straight pin in through the canal to hold it in place to keep it from falling over during the shipping process.

3. When the glue is dry (check dry time on the glue or cement that you are using), place the inside liner back into the shipping box, making sure that the impression is not touching the walls of the impression box at all. Generally, two powder-and-liquid impressions or two silicone impressions can fit in one impression box comfortably. Do not try to ship with more than two impressions, as they are much more likely to get damaged in the shipping process. Do not pack with cotton or tissue and do not place anything else in the box that could potentially damage the impression.

4. Once the impression is in the box and you have checked that it is not touching the walls of the box, fold the order form and place it inside the flap of the impression box. Then fold the order form over the top of the impression box, making sure that it is not down inside the box where the impressions are. Most impression boxes have this clearly marked and some even offer instructions on how to pack the order form on the impression box.

REFERENCES

Mynders, J. M. (2006). *Custom earmold manual* (8th ed.). Ambridge, PA: Microsonic.

Taylor, B., & Mueller, H. G. (2011). *Fitting and dispensing hearing aids*. San Diego, CA: Plural Publishing.

MODULE 2

Putting It All Together

There is a hands-on section on almost all state examinations for taking ear impressions. The way each state tests this section may vary to some degree, so you *must read the information provided by your state* to know what is expected of you. What does remain fairly constant is the way in which *you* go about the process of taking the impression, so that is what is presented here.

States may have you bring your own subject, provide a subject for you, or have you take an impression on a rubber ear or a replica head. Whatever the case may be, you need to treat that "subject" as if he/she were a patient in your office.

1. Have all required equipment as stated by your state in a clear plastic bag.
2. Sanitize hands before beginning.
3. Remove your clean white towel from your bag and place it on the table. This will be your sanitary area to place all of your sanitized equipment.
4. When removing your equipment from your bag, sanitize everything before laying it out on the towel. Set up the equipment in the order in which you will be using it to ensure that you do not skip any steps. The order should be as follows (Figure M2–1):

   a. Otoscope with two speculum tips
   b. Otolight
   c. Otoblocks of various sizes
   d. Another speculum tip (mainly as a reminder to check the block placement, not necessarily to use as you will have the tip still on your otoscope)
   e. Two impression syringes or one impression gun, if allowed by the state

f. Enough impression material for two ear impressions
g. Another speculum tip (mainly as a reminder to check the ear after removing the impression)

5. Place patients in the provided chair at an angle at which you can easily access both ears to take an impression.
6. Instruct patients that you are going to be examining their ear canals and then ask the eight FDA questions if required by your state:

   a. State that you will be examining the outer ear for any visible deformity either congenital or traumatic.
   b. Do they have a history of active drainage from the ear in the past 90 days?
   c. Have they experienced acute or chronic dizziness in the past 90 days?
   d. Have they ever been told that they have a conductive hearing loss? (audiometric air–bone gap greater than or equal to 15 dB at 500 Hz, 1000 Hz, and 2000 Hz).
   e. Have they ever had cerumen removed from their ears? (You can also let the patient know that you will be looking for any visible signs of cerumen during your otoscopic exam.)
   f. Do they experience a hearing loss in only one ear (unilateral hearing loss)?
   g. Have they experienced a sudden hearing loss in one or both ears in the past 90 days?
   h. Do they experience any pain or discomfort in their ears?

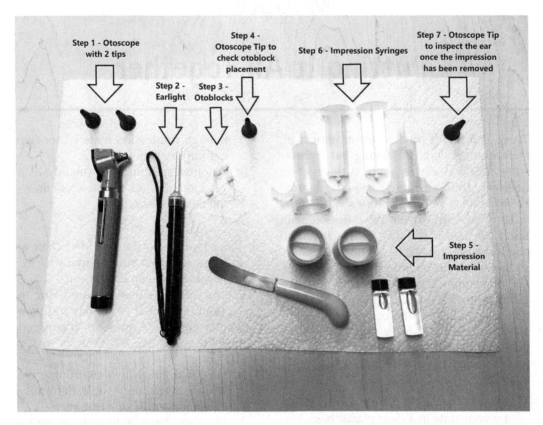

Figure M2–1. The order of supplies used to take an ear impression. Place everything in the order in which you will use it.

7. Instruct the patient on what you are going to do. For example: "I will be taking an ear impression of your ear. I will first inspect your ears with my otoscope to ensure that everything looks good to proceed. Then I will place a cotton/foam block in your ear canal and then inject the material into your ear canal. The material will take about 10 to 12 minutes to set up (check with exact setup time of your particular material) in which time you may not hear anything from that ear/ears. Do you have any questions before we begin?"

8. Sanitize your hands again before you begin. With the otoscope, inspect the outer ear for any abnormalities before proceeding to inspect inside the ear.

Explain out loud to the proctors what you are doing and seeing during your otoscopic inspection. Ensure that you are using the proper bridge-and-brace technique (see Chapter 5) to ensure patient safety. Be sure that you are using a separate otoscope tip for each ear. While inspecting the ear, you can describe to the proctors what you are seeing. For example: "I see the canal walls, which are clear and free of wax. I can see the first bend and the second bend of the canal. I can see the eardrum and the cone of light reflecting back from the light source."

9. Choose the correct-size otoblock to place in the patient's ear canal. (If you are using your own subject, you should already

know what size otoblock you need to use to ensure that a safe impression can be taken.) You cannot touch the cotton when inserting it in the ear (Figure M2–2 shows proper insertion). Once the cotton is placed in the bowl of the ear, use your ear-light to insert the otoblock properly in the ear canal using the bridge-and-brace technique by gently guiding the otoblock into the patient's ear canal.

10. Once you have the otoblock in place, reinspect the ear to ensure that the block is fully blocking the ear canal and you cannot see any gaps between the otoblock and the canal wall where the impression material could pass. Start with your otoscope at the 12 o'clock position and then slowly go in a clockwise direction around the entire circumference of the canal to ensure that you have checked the entire block. Once you have checked the placement, the proctors will check the placement as well and let you know whether or not it is safe to proceed with the impression.

11. Now it is time for you to mix your impression material. (Note: Read all the information that your state sends you about impression materials. Many states do not allow impression guns to be used during the exam, and others do not allow you to mix materials using your bare hands. If you are unsure, contact your state board.)

12. After mixing the impression material, load it into your syringe. Be sure to test the material for consistency and ensure that you do not have air pockets in the syringe. Inject the material into the ear canal using the proper bridge-and-brace technique. Start at the area in between the tragus and the antitragus and insert the tip of the syringe into the canal and inject the material into the canal until you see the material coming back out at you. Then start to move the syringe tip out of the canal and fill up the concha bowl, then work your way

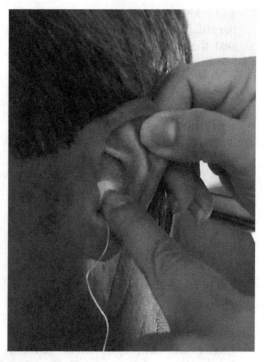

Figure M2–2. Proper placement of the otoblock ensuring sanitary precautions.

up to the helix, fill the helix area, and then return back down to the tragus area. Do not pack the material into the ear as this will cause the impression to distort. Let the material set for at least the allotted time per the manufacturer directions.

13. While the impression material is curing, reclean your equipment and place it back in your bag leaving out your otoscope and clean otoscope tips.

14. Keep time on the wall clock or timer.

15. When it is time to remove the impression, sanitize your hands before touching the impression. (Note: In most states you cannot do the fingernail test of the impression to see if the impression material is cured, you *must* go by time.)

16. Carefully remove the impression from the ear canal. Be sure to loosen the impression by moving the pinna around

and asking the patient to open and close her/his mouth in order to break the seal that may have been formed during the impression. Then start to pull the impression out of the helix area of the ear first. Once it is pulled out of the helix, slowly pull the impression and rotate it toward the patient's nose until it is completely out of the ear.

17. Once the impression is removed, place it on the towel, and *reinspect the ear canal* using the proper bridge-and-brace technique telling the proctor that you are checking to ensure that all the material was removed and state that the ear is clear.

18. You may be required by the state to tell the proctor about the impression (see Chapter 12). Is the impression smooth and complete? Did the impression material meet the otoblock at a flat angle? Is the helix area shown clearly? Were the tragus and antitragus areas covered by the impression material? Can they be clearly defined and seen? You may be asked by the state to point out these landmarks on the impression. If the impression is not perfect, tell the proctor this and state that you would take another one and not send this one to the manufacturer.

19. If there is an impression box present, explain to the proctor how you would package the impression along with the paperwork. Glue the impression down to the bottom of the impression box if you are using powder-and-liquid impression material. You would ensure that the paperwork would be slipped into the side of the box so as to not have it make contact with the impression.

20. You may also be asked by your state to perform other tasks while the impression is curing; for example, look at pictures of ear canals and be asked to identify if they are suitable for ear impressions or not.

Congratulations, you have now completed the impression-taking section of the state licensing exam!

MODULE 2 TEST QUESTIONS

1. Which of the following is true about bridging and bracing?
   a. It is not important
   b. It is not necessary if you know the patient
   c. It should be performed with every patient every time
   d. None of the above

2. It is not important to break the seal of the impression before removing it from the patient's ear.
   a. True
   b. False

3. It is important to wash your hands:
   a. Before touching the patient
   b. Before setting up your equipment
   c. After touching the ear impression
   d. All of the above

4. It is common practice to use one speculum tip to inspect both ear canals.
   a. True
   b. False

5. Immediately after the ear impression is removed from the ear you should:
   a. Tell the proctor you are done and clean up
   b. Tell the proctor it is a good or bad impression
   c. Describe the landmarks of the impression to the proctor
   d. Put the impression down and reinspect the ear canal

6. An otoscopic inspection of the ear is only important the first time you see the patient.
   a. True
   b. False

7. How much time should you allow for the impression material to set up?
   a. As long as it takes
   b. When you test it with you finger and it feels set up
   c. According to the manufacturers set up time
   d. All of the above

8. It is not important to instruct the patient on what you will be doing when taking an impression.
   a. True
   b. False

9. It is important to clean your hands before handling the otoblock.
   a. True
   b. False

10. To ensure proper placement of the otoblock you should:
    a. Place the block a quarter-inch past the second bend
    b. Make sure there are no gaps around the otoblock
    c. Make sure the placement yields sufficient canal length
    d. All of the above

For more quiz questions for Module 2, visit the companion website and test your knowledge.

MODULE 3

Hearing Instrument Fitting and Orientation

13

Delivering a Behind-the-Ear Hearing Aid or Receiver-in-the-Canal Hearing Aid

Objectives

- To prepare the candidate to demonstrate the process of a predelivery check of a behind-the-ear hearing aid (BTE) and receiver-in-the-canal hearing aid (RIC)
- To prepare the candidate to demonstrate the process of delivery of a BTE/RIC on a patient
- To prepare the candidate to understand the basic operation and function of a BTE/RIC

Hearing instruments have evolved immensely over the years, and because of this, the technology that goes into the building and fitting of hearing aids has become more advanced. Due to the advancement in technology and the fact that there are multiple manufacturers that each have their own fitting software and terms for the features equipped in the aids, most states have stuck with the basics when it comes to the hearing aid sections of the practical exam, because to incorporate digital programmable aids into the testing would involve too many variables, since the technology in the hearing aids is not consistent from one manufacturer to another.

In this chapter as well as in Chapter 15, we cover the basics when it comes to hearing aids, because to understand the more advanced technology and features, you first need to master the basics. So for the purpose of this chapter, we focus on the basic components of the BTE (Figure 13–1) and RIC (Figure 13–2) style hearing aids.

PREDELIVERY INSPECTION

Predelivery inspection is done before the patient comes in for the initial fitting. This chapter focuses on the general process of the predelivery inspection, and at the end of this module, in the "Putting It All Together" section, you will find the step-by-step procedures to follow for your state licensing examination. For the predelivery inspection section of your exam, you will be talking out loud to the proctors and pretending that you are going through your predelivery routine. Talk out loud and explain everything that you would do even if you are not actually asked to perform it during your exam. Start by stating, "In our office we do a predelivery inspection on all hearing instruments prior to the patient coming in for the delivery. This process allows us to check the BTE or RIC instrument and custom earmold against our order form and to check to make sure the features and options are working properly and that the devices that we received are as we ordered them. We then perform a listening check on the device as well as run a 2-cc coupler measurement, preset the programming, and/or ensure switches and controls are in working order and are set according to

User Switch   Earhook

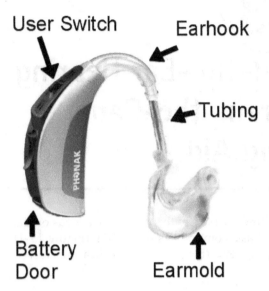

←Tubing

Battery
Door   Earmold

Figure 13–1. Basic external components and features of a BTE style hearing aid with tubing and custom earmold. (Photos courtesy of Phonak and Westone)

the patient's hearing loss and MCL/UCL measurements."

↝ During the predelivery inspection you want to make sure that you have a copy of your order forms (for both the hearing instrument and the custom earmold order), the hearing instrument BTE/RIC spec sheet from the manufacturer, as well as the earmold invoice and manufacturer invoice for the hearing device. State that you will be checking the hearing instrument against the patient's record for degree of hearing loss as well as the patient's most comfortable hearing level (MCL), uncomfortable hearing level (UCL), and lifestyle to confirm that the instruments ordered for the patient are appropriate. Ensure that it is the correct color that you ordered and that it has all the options that you ordered. For a BTE be sure to check the earhook and filters. For RIC, check the receiver side (right or left), power (output and gain of the receiver), and length of the device. When inspecting the earmold, ensure that the color, venting, and tubing are appropriate and what you ordered. Check to make sure that

there are no rough edges on the earmold by rubbing the earmold on your forearm; make sure the earmold feels smooth.

LISTENING CHECK

Perform a listening check of the device to make sure that it is functioning up to specifications. You do so by carrying out the following steps:

1. Install the battery and open and close the door multiple times.
↝ 2. Check the volume control taper (if applicable).
3. Check the controls (if applicable) or read out the best-fit program if the aid is a programmable device and ensure that you are able to read the aids in the manufacturer's software.
4. Check the memory button (if applicable).
5. Check the telecoil (if applicable).
6. Run a 2-cc coupler measurement using a hearing aid analyzer.

Once the hearing instrument has been inspected and you have determined that it is functioning up to the manufacturer's specifications and that the order was correct, preset the controls or preprogram the instrument based on the patient's audiogram in the manufacturer's software, and then call the patient to come in for the delivery. (Changing earmold tubing is covered in depth in Chapter 16.)

FITTING AND COUNSELING

You are now ready to proceed with the hearing instrument fitting and counseling. As always, sanitize your work area and your hands before touching the patient or the instruments. During your practical exam, you will more than likely be fitting a model (rubber) ear and you are expected to treat

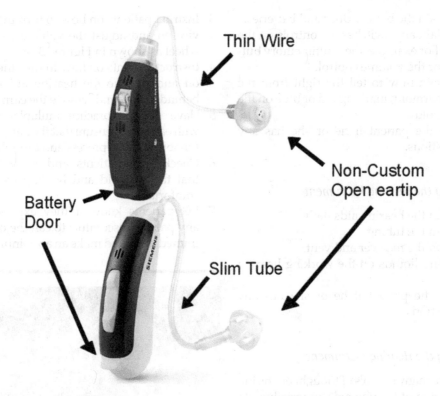

Figure 13–2. Example of an RIC style hearing aid. (From Mueller, Ricketts, & Bentler, 2013, p. 253)

this model ear as if it is a real patient. You should perform an otoscopic inspection of the outer ear and ear canal before proceeding with the fitting. If there is no otoscope or ear light at this particular station during your exam, pretend that you are performing the inspection on the model ear.

The following is the process of fitting and counseling, which is covered in depth at the end of this module.

Introduction to the BTE Hearing Instrument

1. Wash your hands.
2. Wipe the earmold clean.

3. Put the hearing aid behind the patient's ear and insert the earmold in the model/patient's ear.
4. Measure the tubing to the ear-hook and then mark the tubing with a black marker and remove the earmold before cutting the tubing.
5. Remove the hearing aid from the model/patient's ear and attach the earmold tubing to the ear-hook.
6. Fit the earmold and hearing aid back onto the model/patient's ear and ensure that the fit is correct.
7. Explain with the model ear how the earmold fits inside and the BTE fits behind the ear.
8. Remove the earmold and hearing aid from the patient's ear.

9. Explain the battery door and batteries.
10. Explain any switches or controls on the aid. For example, the multimemory button or the volume control.
11. Explain how to tell the right from the left earmold, marking red or blue on the earmolds.
12. Ask the patient if he or she has any questions.

Cleaning the Hearing Instrument

1. Clean the hearing aids daily.
2. Clean the tubing.
3. Clean the receiver and vent.
4. Put no liquids on the working hearing aids.
5. Ask the patient if he or she has any questions.

Wearing the Hearing Instrument

There are many schools of thought on the initial wearing of hearing aids, especially with new hearing aid users, so state something as simple as, "I would encourage patients to wear their hearing instruments as much or as little as they feel comfortable." You could also say that you would put them on a wearing schedule for the first month with follow-up visits to your office on a weekly basis in order to check their progress. Start them with 2 hr in the morning and 2 hr in the evening only at home until they are confident with those 4 hr, and then they can increase their wearing time.

Insertion and Removal of the Hearing Instrument and Earmold

1. To show patients how to insert the earmold inside the ear, start by holding the earmold between your thumb and index finger with the canal portion on the bottom, pointing down toward the canal as shown in Figure 13–3.
2. Insert the earmold and place the BTE behind your ear.

3. Instruct patients on how to turn the device on and adjust the volume control wheel as shown in Figure 13–4.
4. Instruct patients on how to turn the aid off and remove the hearing aid from behind the ear and remove the earmold.
5. Have patients practice multiple times with each ear to ensure that they are comfortable with the process and procedure.
6. Check with patients and make sure that the earmold and hearing aid are comfortable.
7. Let patients know if they experience any pain or discomfort to call the office immediately and make an appointment.

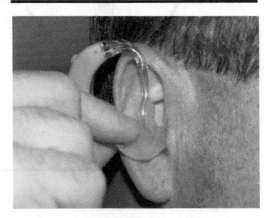

Figure 13–3. An example of how to hold the earmold for insertion.

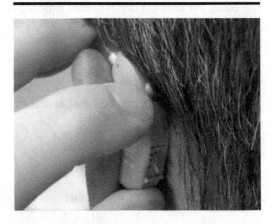

Figure 13–4. An example of how to hold the aid to manipulate the controls.

Verifying the Fit of the Hearing Instrument

1. The hearing instrument should be turned on and the volume control turned on to a comfortable level for listening.
2. You can do a sound-field measurement, speech mapping, or real-ear verification to be sure the fitting adjustments are correct.

Caring for the Hearing Instruments

1. Show the patient how to insert and remove the hearing aid.
2. Show the patient how to use the options such as the telecoil.
3. Show the patient how to insert and remove the battery and what type of battery to use.
4. Show the patient how to use the volume control and the care of the earmold.
5. Instruct the patient to clean the earmold every night before putting it away.
6. Instruct the patient on using the appropriate cleaning tools and how to wipe off the hearing aid and what to use.
7. Inform the patient that the hearing aid must not get wet (e.g., the patient must remove the hearing aid when showering, swimming, or washing his/her hair).
8. Instruct the patient to open the battery door at night or when the hearing aid is not in use.
9. Instruct the patient to discard weak or dead batteries.

Introduction to the RIC Hearing Instrument

1. Wash your hands.
2. Wipe the hearing aid (processor) to ensure it is clean.
3. Put the hearing aid (processor) behind the patient's ear and insert the receiver in the model/patient's ear.
4. Make sure that the receiver length is correct.

5. Explain with the model ear how the receiver and earbud fits inside and the hearing aid processor fits behind the ear.
6. Remove the receiver and hearing aid from the patient's ear.
7. Explain the battery door and batteries.
8. Explain any switches or controls on the aid. For example, the multimemory or the volume control.
9. Explain how to tell the right from the left.
10. Ask the patient if he/she has any questions.

Cleaning the Hearing Instrument

1. Clean the hearing aid daily by wiping it down with a dry cloth.
2. Clean the earbud by brushing it off with the cleaning brush.
3. Put no liquids on the working hearing aids.
4. Ask the patient if he/she has any questions.

Wearing the Hearing Instrument

There are many schools of thought on the initial wearing of hearing aids, especially with new hearing aid users, so state something as simple as, "I would encourage patients to wear their hearing instruments as much or as little as they feel comfortable." You could also say that you would put them on a wearing schedule for the first month with follow-up visits to your office on a weekly basis in order to check their progress. Start them with 2 hr in the morning and 2 hr in the evening only at home until they are confident with those 4 hr, and then they can increase their wearing time.

Insertion and Removal of the Hearing Instrument and Earmold

1. To show patients how to insert the earbud and receiver inside the ear, start by holding the earbud between your thumb

and index finger with the canal portion on the bottom, pointing down toward the canal as shown in Figure 13–5.

2. Insert the earbud and place the hearing aid behind your ear.
3. Instruct patients on how to turn the device on and adjust the volume control wheel as shown in Figure 13–6.
4. Instruct patients on how to turn the aid off (if applicable) and remove the hearing aid from behind the ear and remove the earbud/receiver.
5. Have patients practice multiple times with each ear to ensure that they are comfortable with the process and procedure.
6. Check with patients and make sure that the earbud and hearing aid are comfortable.
7. Let patients know if they experience any pain or discomfort to call the office immediately and make an appointment.

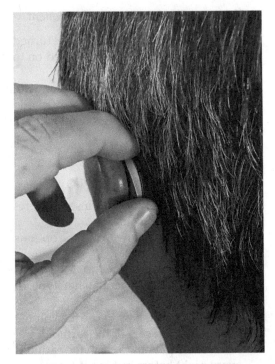

Figure 13–6. An example of how to hold the aid to manipulate the controls.

COUNSELING AND REALISTIC EXPECTATIONS

State that you would have the patient bring a family member to the fitting so that the family member is part of the rehabilitation process and is aware of what the expectations are. The following are examples of some of the things that you can tell the patient and the family member during the initial fitting. Make sure you are comfortable and able to say them out loud in your own words, as this will be part of the initial fitting process on your practical examination.

- Your own voice will sound different to you but should be acceptable.
- Practice reading out loud to yourself to become more accustomed to your own voice.

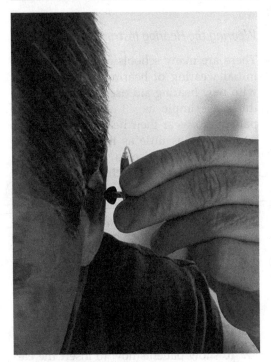

Figure 13–5. An example of how to hold the earbud for insertion.

- Your hearing aids will not restore your hearing to "normal" or what it was when you were younger.
- Have your family and friends get your attention before speaking to you.
- Ask your friends and family to speak quieter to you now; they do not need to yell anymore now that you have your hearing aids.
- Your hearing aids and earmold should fit comfortably and snug.
- When the earmolds and hearing aids are inserted properly, there should not be any feedback.
- Soft speech should be audible, average speech should be comfortable, and loud speech should be loud but comfortable.
- You will be aware of soft sounds that previously were not audible, such as footsteps, the refrigerator, the air conditioner, fans, and so forth.
- To adjust to the volume of your hearing aids, have a friend or family member read to you or ask you questions and practice

repeating what this person says. This will help with your confidence at adjusting and acclimating to your hearing aids.

Regarding paperwork, do the following:

1. Fill out and review with the patient the purchase agreement and trial period (for your state).
2. Fill out and review with the patient the warranty card and policy.
3. Review the instruction manual with the patient and encourage her/him to read it over and call with any questions.
4. Make follow-up appointments and give the appointment card(s) to the patient.
5. It is helpful to have a "delivery folder" for the patient to keep all of this information in so that it is all in one place and can be accessed easily.

REFERENCE

Mueller, H. G., Ricketts, T. A., & Bentler, R. (2013). *Modern hearing aids: Pre-fitting and selection considerations*. San Diego, CA: Plural Publishing.

(14)
Earmolds

Objectives

- To prepare the candidate to choose the proper earmold based on the hearing loss and patient needs
- To prepare the candidate to be knowledgeable about different types of materials used for earmolds
- To prepare the candidate to be knowledgeable about the different types of earmolds and their acoustic options

TERMS AND DEFINITIONS

Damping: the decrease in amplitude of the acoustic signal across the frequency range (can be accomplished by using filters, lamb's wool, or dampers)

Earmold: a custom-made earpiece that fits in the external canal to conduct amplified sound from the receiver of the hearing aid to the tympanic membrane

Sound bore: the hole made in the earmold that holds the tubing and allows for the passage of amplified sound into the ear

Vent: the hole made in an earmold that allows for the passage of air and sounds to reach the tympanic membrane

Please refer to the glossary at the end of this book for more terms and definitions.

EARMOLD SELECTION

The earmold is a very important part of the coupling of a behind-the-ear (BTE) hearing aid to the patient's ear. It not only serves as a coupler but it also serves as part of the acoustic system, and its purpose is to conduct the amplified response from the hearing aid to the tympanic membrane and the rest of the auditory system. There are two main considerations when it comes to choosing and fitting earmolds: the cosmetics of the earmold (the part that holds the hearing aid in place) and the acoustics of the earmold.

The types and styles of earmolds were given standardized names for their physical appearance by the National Association of Earmold Labs (NAEL) in 1970. Names for the earmolds do vary from manufacturer to manufacturer, but generally for the common style of earmolds their names appear somewhat the same. For most state examinations you will need to know what type of earmold you would fit to various hearing losses as well as the acoustic characteristics, and modifications that can be made to the earmolds to achieve a particular response from that earmold and hearing device.

There are many considerations to take into account when it comes to choosing and fitting a custom earmold. As discussed in previous chapters, the type, degree, and configuration of a patient's hearing loss comes into play, as well as the patient's needs, anatomy of the ear, and the dexterity of the patient. All of these factors come into consideration with regard to how you make your choice as to what earmolds you are going to fit. In order to choose the appropriate earmold, let us first start with the patient's ear.

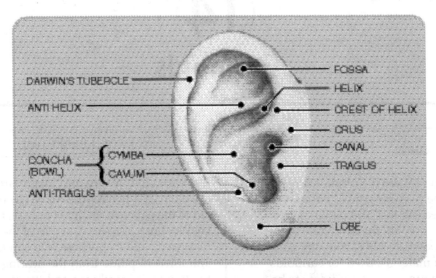

Figure 14–1. Anatomy of the outer ear. (From Mynders, 2006)

Figure 14–1 points out all of the landmarks of a healthy pinna. Before discussing a particular earmold with a patient, you must evaluate the patient's ear and make sure that the earmold that you are considering is appropriate for that ear. Evaluate the pinna and the skin and ask yourself if it is soft, medium, or hard. Does the skin appear thin? Will a harder material be difficult to insert into this ear if the texture of the ear is hard? Do all the landmarks of the patient's ear appear normal? Will anything about this ear cause concern with the fit and with insertion and removal?

Next, you want to consider the patient's type, degree, and configuration of hearing loss, as well as the matrix of the hearing aid that you are going to be fitting on the earmold. There are many different earmolds for different types of losses, and unfortunately, as stated previously, there are no "true" names for types or styles of earmolds, but we discuss the common ones and their accepted names later in this chapter (Table 14–1). Figure 14–2 is a drawing of three basic types of earmolds and their relationship to the human ear as shown in Figure 14–1. You can get a good idea of the fit of the earmold and how it will fit in the ear by reviewing these two figures.

The purpose of this chapter is not to teach you everything there is to know about earmolds but to review the important concepts and aspects of earmolds for the purpose of applying the information for the practical portion of your state exam. Much of this should be review for you, as you should have already studied earmolds for the written portion of your state exam, but

Table 14–1. Severity of Hearing Loss

Earmold Style	Mild	Moderate	Severe to Profound
Receiver		✓	✓
Standard	✓	✓	✓
Skeleton	✓	✓	✓
Semiskeleton	✓	✓	
Canal/canal lock	✓	✓	
Nonoccluding	✓	✓	

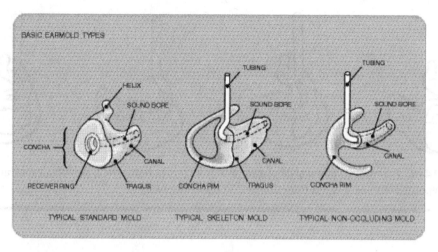

Figure 14–2. Common key landmarks of the various types of earmolds. (From Mynders, 2006)

if this is not a review, you may want to read and study more in-depth literature on earmolds before continuing with this chapter (see References).

STYLE OPTIONS

Style options are as follows:

- *Standard* (regular). This is the most problem-free earmold and is used when the acoustic seal is a major factor in achieving an effective hearing aid fitting, particularly in the application of high-gain instruments (Figure 14–3).
- *Skeleton*. This is the most popular style of earmold. As shown in Figure 14–3, it has an open space in the concha for comfort and appearance. It maintains retention and is a good fit with the outer ring of the concha and helix forming a good seal. This type of earmold is a good choice for mild to moderate hearing losses.

- *Semiskeleton*. Semiskeleton means that a portion or multiple portions of the concha are removed from the standard skeleton earmold. This type of earmold is good to use when the back portion of the concha is "flat" and does not give any extra retention, although the more retention you have, the better the acoustic seal is.
- *Canal lock*. This type of earmold was developed for people who preferred the canal-style earmold but may have abnormalities of the ear that prevent a good retention. The canal lock has a fingerlike projection that runs along the bottom of the concha area that acts as a lock to hold the canal portion of the earmold in place.
- *Canal*. It is the same as the canal-lock style without the lock portion. Usually with this type of earmold you need to have a long canal in order to get good retention (Figure 14–3).
- *Free field*. This is an earmold belonging to the nonoccluding

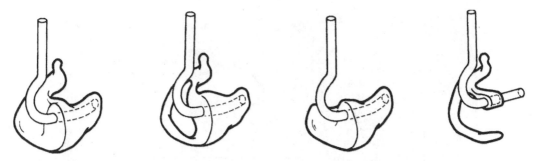

Figure 14–3. The most common style of earmolds from left to right: shell, skeleton, canal, and free-field. (Reprinted with permission from Unitron. All rights reserved)

family. As shown in Figure 14–3, the canal portion of the earmold is at the top of the canal, giving the greatest amount of open space in the aperture of the canal. This earmold is recommended when there is a call to reduce or eliminate frequencies below 1000 Hz.

■ *Receiver earmold.* This style of earmold is used with body-aid hearing aids that have external receivers clipped into the earmold. Regular-style earmolds have connecting rings (0.25-inch standard) that can be vinyl or metal and can usually be made in both hard and soft materials.

EARMOLD MATERIAL

There are many different materials used to build earmolds that may vary among manufacturers. For the purpose of this manual, we discuss only the most common types of materials and their characteristics, as well as the types of hearing loss for which they should be fit. Due to the fact that there are many different earmold manufacturers, each of which chooses to name its materials dif-

ferently, we refer to the various materials by their chemical names and in parentheses we list some common manufacturer names.

■ *Poly methyl methacrylate* (lucite, acrylic) is a durable, hard, long-lasting material of fine- and extra-fine-grade dental acrylic to be considered for fitting of mild and moderate losses. It is sometimes a heat cure process which is used for those with allergy issues.

■ *Poly ethyl methacrylate* (Vinylflex II, Starflex) is a soft material that is heat cured and softens with the body's temperature.

■ *Poly methyl methacrylate and polyethyl methacrylate* (flex canal, acrylic body with VinylFlex canal, soft canal) are a combination of both hard and soft materials on the same earmold.

■ *Thermoplastic polyvinyl chloride* (Supersoft, Synth-A-Flex, Ultraflex) is recommended for fitting those with severe hearing losses, as it is a soft and durable material that provides a better acoustic seal.

■ *Silicone* (Medi-Sil II, Emplex, Mediflex) is most often used when there is a severe hearing loss with a power hearing aid. It is a soft material that is also used when a patient presents with an allergy problem.

- *Polyethylene* is a semihard material that is most commonly used in severe allergy cases. Modification of this material is not recommended.

ACOUSTIC OPTIONS

Although there are different styles of earmolds that are used for different types of hearing loss, it is important to know that there are different acoustic options that can be made to those earmolds to accomplish various acoustic changes for both sound quality and appropriateness for the loss. Let us take a look at basic earmold acoustics.

Tubing

All earmolds need some type of tubing to couple them to the BTE hearing aids. The NAEL has standardized 10 tubing sizes, but only 6 of the 10 have a difference in the inside diameter, so those are the ones most commonly used (Mynders, 2006). Table 14–2 summarizes the different tubing sizes with their inside and outside diameters. The tubing sizes that are shown in bold are the sizes that are most commonly used.

It is important to note that the various sizes of tubing can have an effect on the response of the hearing aid. It is not so much the length of the tubing that has minimal effect on the performance of the hearing aid as it is the internal diameter of the tubing. The larger the internal diameter of the tubing, the more increase there is in the high-frequency gain; and the smaller the internal diameter, the more decrease there is in the high-frequency gain.

Table 14–2. Standard Tubing Sizes of the National Association of Earmold Labs

Size/Type	Inside Diameter		Outside Diameter	
9	.094"	2.4 mm	0.160"	4.1 mm
12	.085"	2.2 mm	0.125"	3.2 mm
13 Standard	.076"	1.9 mm	0.116"	2.9 mm
13 Medium	.076"	1.9 mm	0.122"	3.2 mm
13 Thick wall	.076"	1.9 mm	0.130"	3.3 mm
13 Double wall	.076"	1.9 mm	0.142"	3.6 mm
14	.066"	1.7 mm	0.116"	2.9 mm
15	.059"	1.5 mm	0.116"	2.9 mm
16 Standard	.053"	1.3 mm	0.116"	2.9 mm
16 Standard	.053"	1.3 mm	0.116"	2.9 mm
16 Thin	.053"	1.3 mm	.085"	2.2 mm

Venting

There are three types of venting that are generally used with earmolds: parallel, diagonal, and external. A parallel vent is recommended whenever possible, as it runs parallel to the sound bore but does not intersect it. This type of vent generally does not affect the response of the sound as much as a diagonal vent but does affect the low frequencies more than the diagonal vent. A diagonal vent intersects with the sound bore and should do so as close to the end of the bore as possible. This type of vent is used when there is limited space in the canal and there is not enough room for a parallel vent. The last and final vent is the external vent. This type of vent is a grooved channel that is cut along the outside of the earmold and is sometimes referred to as a trench vent. This type of vent is used when there is physically no space to use either the parallel vent or the diagonal vent. (See Figure 14–4 for the different types of venting.) The size of the vent, depending on its length and diameter, can produce minimal to maximum changes in the response of the hearing aid. There are three main reasons that vents are used in earmolds:

1. To increase the comfort to the patient
2. To improve sound quality of the response of the hearing aid
3. To change the response of the hearing aid

Vent sizes can vary slightly from manufacturer to manufacturer, but an approximation of the three most common vent sizes are as follows:

1. Small vent—0.040 inch
2. Medium vent—0.082 inch
3. Large vent—0.128 inch

The effect the vent size has on the response curve primarily changes the response

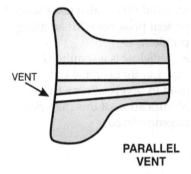

PARALLEL VENT

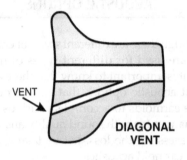

DIAGONAL VENT

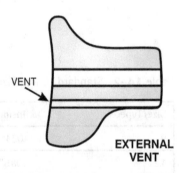

EXTERNAL VENT

Figure 14–4. Parallel, diagonal, and external venting. (From Mynders, 2006)

below 1000 Hz. The larger the vent diameter, the more the low frequencies are decreased. It is important to remember and use caution when choosing venting because it can also cause feedback as well, if you are attempting to provide a lot of gain to the

Table 14–3. Custom Vent Effect

Frequency (Hz)	Diameter		Length	
250	.042"	1.1 mm	0.7"	17.8 mm
250	.030"	0.8 mm	0.35"	8.9 mm
500	.085"	2.2 mm	0.7"	17.8 mm
500	.060"	1.5 mm	0.35"	8.9 mm
500	.042"	1.1 mm	0.175"	4.4 mm
750	0.120"	3.0 mm	0.7"	17.8 mm
750	.090"	2.3 mm	0.35"	8.9 mm
750	.063"	1.6 mm	0.175"	4.4 mm
1000	0.168"	4.3 mm	0.7"	17.8 mm
1000	0.120"	3.0 mm	0.35"	8.9 mm
1000	.084"	2.1 mm	0.175"	4.4 mm
1000	.059"	1.5 mm	.0875"	2.2 mm

high frequencies. See Table 14–3 for vent size and frequency comparison.

Other Acoustic Options

It is important for you to know, but not the main purpose of this manual or chapter, the other acoustic options that can primarily affect the mid-frequency range. (See the works listed in the References for more in-depth information on the effects and use of lamb's wool, filters, and dampers.) You should also be familiar with modifications that can be done to the earmolds themselves such as a bell canal, horn and reverse horn bore, Libby horn, and continuous flow adaptors. Table 14–4 shows many of the adaptations that can be made to earmolds to produce the desired response.

REFERENCES

Mynders, J. M. (2006). *Custom earmold manual* (8th ed.). Ambridge, PA: Microsonic.

Taylor, B., & Mueller, H. G. (2017). *Fitting and dispensing hearing aids* (2nd ed.). San Diego, CA: Plural Publishing.

Table 14–4. Classical Modification and Effects Chart

Modification		Effect on Low Frequencies (Below 750 Hz)	Effect on Frequencies Between 750 and 1500 Hz	Effect on Frequencies Between 1500 and 3000 Hz	Effect on High Frequencies (Above 3000 Hz)
Tubing Diameter	Larger I.D. tubing & horn tubing	Negligible	Moves peak to higher frequency	Increases height of peak and moves to higher frequency	Increases
	Smaller I.D. tubing	May reduce below 1 kHz	Moves peak to lower frequency	Reduces height of peak and moves to lower frequency	Large reduction
Tubing Length	Longer tubing	Increases	Moves peak to lower frequency	Moves peak to lower frequency	Negligible
	Shorter tubing	Slightly decreases	Moves peak to higher frequency	Moves peak to higher frequency	Negligible
Length of Earmold Canal	Longer earmold canal	----------Increases level of response curve----------			
	Shorter earmold canal	----------Decreases level of response curve----------			
Bore Diameter	Larger diameter bore through earmold canal*	Negligible	Moves peak to higher frequency	Moves peak to higher frequency	Increases
	Smaller diameter through earmold canal*	Negligible	Moves peak to lower frequency	Moves peak to lower frequency	Decreases
Bore Length	Longer bore through earmold canal*	Slightly decreases	Moves peak to lower frequency	Moves peak to lower frequency	Decreases
	Shorter bore through earmold canal	Slightly decreases	Moves peak to higher frequency	Moves peak to higher frequency	Increases

Table 14–4. *Continued*

Modification		Effect on Low Frequencies (Below 750 Hz)	Effect on Frequencies Between 750 and 1500 Hz	Effect on Frequencies Between 1500 and 3000 Hz	Effect on High Frequencies (Above 3000 Hz)
Venting	Small vent (.031″/0.8 mm)**	Negligible	Negligible	Negligible	Negligible
	Medium vent (.064″/1.6 mm)**	Decreases	Increases peak heights	Negligible	Negligible
	Large vent (.094″/2.4 mm)**	Decreases	Increases peak heights	Negligible	Negligible
Non-occluding Earmold	Non-occluding earmold	Eliminates	Moves peak to higher frequency and increases height	Increases peak height	Negligible
Open Vent Earmold	Open-vented (high frequency earmold)	Decreases	Reduces peak height	Negligible	Negligible
Filter Inserts	Filter insert at hearing aid nub	Negligible	Reduces peak height	Reduces peak height	Negligible
	Filter insert at earmold tip	Slightly decreases	Large reduction	Large reduction	Decreases

Note. Because of wide variation in earphone types and internal acoustical systems in hearing aids, this chart must be considered as a guide for average conditions.

* Applies to earmolds for conventional earphones.

** Vents of short length are more effective in reducing low frequency response. Gain must be limited with larger size vents to avoid feedback. Reprinted with permission by Microsonic.

15

Delivering an In–the–Ear Hearing Aid

Objectives

- To prepare the candidate to demonstrate the process of a predelivery check of an in-the-ear hearing aid (ITE)
- To prepare the candidate to demonstrate the process of delivery of an ITE on a patient
- To prepare the candidate to understand the basic operation and function of an ITE

As stated in Chapter 13, due to the evolution of hearing aid technology and the multiple factors that go into the fitting and programming of modern hearing aids, we focus only on the largest of the custom styles commonly referred to as an in-the-ear hearing aid (ITE), but the information in this chapter can be applied to any custom hearing aids that you may be tested on during the practical portion of your state exam, including in-the-canal hearing aids (ITCs) and completely in-the-canal hearing aids (CICs) (Figure 15–1).

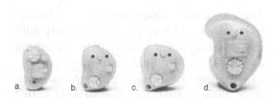

a.   b.   c.   d.

Figure 15–1. Examples of four traditions of custom hearing aid styles.

Predelivery inspection is done before the patient comes in for the initial fitting. This chapter focuses on the general process of the predelivery inspection, and at the end of this module you will find the step-by-step procedures to follow for your state licensing examination. For the predelivery inspection of the ITE you will be talking out loud to the proctors and pretending that you are going through your routine. Explain everything that you would do even if you are not actually asked to perform it during your exam. Start by stating, "In our office we do a predelivery inspection on all hearing instruments prior to the patient coming in for the delivery. This process allows us to check the ITE instrument against our order form and to check to make sure the features and options are working properly and devices we received are as we ordered them. We will then perform a listening check on the device as well as run a 2-cc coupler measurement and preset the programming, and/or ensure switches are in working order and they are set according to the patient's hearing loss and MCL/UCL measurements."

During the predelivery inspection you want to make sure that you have your order form and the manufacturer invoice for the hearing device. State that you will be checking the hearing instrument against the degree of hearing loss as well as the patient's most comfortable hearing level (MCL), uncomfortable hearing level (UCL), and lifestyle to confirm that the instruments ordered for the patient are appropriate. Ensure that it is the correct color that you ordered and that is has all the options that you ordered. Check to make sure that there are no rough edges on the canal and helix portion of the hearing instrument by rubbing the instruments on your forearm, making sure those areas are smooth.

LISTENING CHECK

Perform a listening check of the device to make sure that it is functioning up to specifications. You do so by carrying out the following steps:

1. Insert the battery and open and close the door multiple times.
2. Check the volume control taper (if applicable).
3. Check the controls (if applicable) or read out the best-fit program if the aid is a programmable device and ensure that you are able to read the aids in the manufacturer's software.
4. Check the memory buttons (if applicable).
5. Check the telecoil (if applicable).
6. Run 2-cc coupler measurement.

Once the hearing instrument has been inspected and you have determined that it is functioning up to the manufacturer's specifications and that the order was correct, preset the trimmer controls based on the patient's audiogram, and then call the patient to come in for the delivery.

FITTING AND COUNSELING

You are now ready to proceed with the hearing instrument fitting and counseling. As always, you must sanitize your work area and your hands before touching the patient or the instruments. During your state exam, you will more than likely be fitting a model

(rubber) ear and you are to treat this model ear as if it is a real patient. You should perform an otoscopic inspection of the outer ear and ear canal before proceeding with the fitting. If there is no otoscope or earlight at this particular station during your exam, pretend that you are doing it on the model ear.

The following is the process of fitting and counseling, which is covered in depth at the end of this module.

Introduction to the Hearing Instrument

1. Wash your hands.
2. Wipe the hearing aid clean with a sanitary cloth.
3. Explain with the model ear how the ITE fits inside the ear.
4. Explain the battery door and batteries.
5. Explain any switches on the aid.
6. Demonstrate the volume control.
7. Explain how to tell the right from the left hearing aid, the red and blue indicators.
8. Ask the patient if he or she has any questions.

Cleaning the Hearing Instrument

1. Clean the hearing aids daily.
2. Clean the receiver and vent.
3. No liquids are to be used on the hearing aids.
4. Ask the patient if he or she has any questions.

Wearing the Hearing Instrument

There are many schools of thought on the initial wearing of hearing aids, especially with new hearing aid users, so state something as simple as "I would encourage patients to wear their hearing instruments as much or as little as they feel comfortable with." You could also say that you would put them on a wearing schedule for the first month with follow-up visits to your office on a weekly basis in order to check on their progress. Start them with 2 hr in the morning and 2 hr in the evening only at home until they are confident with those 4 hr, and then they can increase their wearing time.

Insertion and Removal of the Hearing Instrument

1. To show the patient how to insert the hearing aid inside the ear, start by holding the hearing aid between your thumb and forefinger.
2. Insert the canal portion, and using a twisting motion work the hearing aid into the ear.
3. Gently rotate the hearing aid into the bowl portion of the ear and then pull down on your earlobe and insert the instrument firmly into place.
4. Instruct patients on how to turn the device on and adjust the volume control wheel.
5. To remove the hearing instrument, turn the volume control off by rotating it toward the back of your head.
6. Grab the instrument with your thumb and forefinger and rotate the aid toward your nose while gently pulling it out.

Verifying the Fit of the Hearing Instrument

1. The ITE volume control should be turned on to a comfortable level for listening by rotating the volume control wheel toward your nose.
2. You can do a sound-field measurement, speech mapping measurement, or real-ear verification to be sure the fitting adjustments are correct.

Caring for the Hearing Instruments

1. Show the patient how to insert and remove the hearing aid.
2. Show the patient how to use the options such as the telecoil.

3. Show the patient how to insert and remove the battery and what type of battery to use.
4. Show the patient how to use the volume control.
5. Instruct the patient to clean the hearing aid every night before putting it away.
6. Instruct the patient on using the appropriate cleaning tools and how to wipe off the hearing aid and what to use.
7. Inform the patient that the hearing aid must not get wet (e.g., the patient must remove the hearing aid when showering, swimming, or washing his/her hair).
8. Instruct the patient to open the battery door at night or when the hearing aid is not in use.
9. Instruct the patient to discard weak or dead batteries.

COUNSELING AND REALISTIC EXPECTATIONS

State that you would have the patient bring a family member to the fitting so that the family member is part of the rehabilitation process and is aware of what the expectations are. The following are examples of some of the things that you can tell the patient and the family member during the initial fitting. Make sure you are comfortable and able to say them out loud in your own words, as this will be part of the initial fitting process on your practical examination.

- Your own voice will sound different to you but should be acceptable.
- Practice reading out loud to yourself to become more accustomed to your own voice.
- Your hearing aids will not restore your hearing to "normal" or what it was when you were younger.
- Have your family and friends get your attention before speaking to you.

- Ask your friends and family to speak quieter to you now; they do not need to yell anymore now that you have your hearing aids.
- Your hearing aids should fit comfortably and snug.
- When the hearing aids are inserted properly, there should not be any feedback.
- Soft speech should be audible, average speech should be comfortable, and loud speech should be loud but comfortable.
- You will be aware of soft sounds that previously were not audible, such as footsteps, the refrigerator, the air conditioner, fans, and so forth.
- To adjust to the volume of your hearing aids, have a friend or family member read to you or ask you questions and practice repeating what they say. This will help with your confidence at adjusting and acclimating to your hearing aids.

Regarding paperwork, do the following:

1. Fill out and review with the patient the purchase agreement and trial period (for your state).
2. Fill out and review with the patient the warranty card and policy.
3. Review the instruction manual with the patient and encourage the patient to read it over and call with any questions.
4. Make follow-up appointments and give the appointment card(s) to the patient.
5. It is helpful to have a "delivery folder" for the patient to keep all of this information in so that it is all in one place and can be accessed easily.

MODULE 3

Putting It All Together

On most state examinations you will be evaluated on the fitting of new hearing aids, mainly behind-the-ear (BTE) and in-the-ear (ITE) styles that are generally *not* programmable or digital hearing aids. It is very costly for states to rewrite exams, and for that reason, most states are still testing using BTE and ITE style aids that have manual volume control wheels and trimmer controls on them. You will usually only need to bring a stethoscope or other listening device to this portion of the examination and the rest of the supplies will be provided for you. Ensure that you read the information provided to you by the state to know exactly what is expected of you. Be cognizant of how much time you are allotted for this particular section, as you will need to practice the fitting and delivery process and get it all completed in the amount of time that they give you. You will not have an hour like you would in your office to complete this process, so it is important that you know and can verbalize the step-by-step process so you are well prepared for your practical exam.

For most states you will not have a patient there to deliver the hearing aids to, so the model ear that is provided to you *is* your patient for that section. Treat that ear as if it were your patient's ear and talk out loud when you go through the process of the predelivery and fitting of the hearing instrument. I have provided a brief 16-step process for the fitting and delivery of an ITE, BTE, and RIC hearing aid. Use this process as a guideline, adding to it as you practice to make sure you are touching on all the important aspects of this portion of your exam. After the 16-step process, you will find additional information that you can add to make the fitting and delivery process your own.

DELIVERY OF AN ITE HEARING AID

1. Predelivery of the ITE: State out loud, "In our office, we first wash our hands before handling any hearing aid. The model, size, serial numbers, specifications, battery size, and color are checked against the order form and patient record. A listening check is performed and any needed adjustments are made to the devices prior to delivery. The battery compartment, microphone, receiver, vent, and all movable parts are checked and inspected. I also rub the hearing aid on my forearm checking to see if there are any sharp edges. I also run a 2-cc coupler measurement to ensure that the hearing aids are up to specifications according to the manufacturer's spec sheet."

2. Listening check: "I always check the contacts of the battery and ensure that the battery fits properly and that the battery door opens and closes with ease. The volume control is checked to make sure I can hear it getting louder and softer and that there is no static or intermittency. Everything appears to be in order."

3. Predelivery adjustments: "The hearing aids are always checked against the patient's audiogram, MCL, and UCL. We make sure that the hearing aid can be read in the manufacturer software and is best-fit accordingly while listening to the hearing aids."

4. Fitting and delivery of the ITE: "I have completed the predelivery inspection, listening check, and adjustments. During the delivery process I go over many points in detail with my patient We also run real-ear measurements on every patient to help with verification and adjustments of the fitting during the delivery process."

5. Otoscopic inspection: "I perform an otoscopic inspection of the pinna and canal prior to the delivery of the hearing aids."

6. Expectations: "I guide the patient through what to expect and what not to expect from the hearing aids."

7. Family: "I encourage the family to participate in the hearing aid fitting."

8. Introduction: "I wash my hands before starting the fitting and delivery process."

9. Cleaning: "I instruct patients on the proper cleaning techniques and have them demonstrate them to me so I can ensure that they understand how to clean the instruments properly."

10. Wearing: "Patients are instructed to wear the hearing aids as much as possible or as much as they feel comfortable. In my office, we give the patient a 2- to 3-week rehabilitation program to follow and regularly scheduled appointments."

11. Feedback: "Feedback is explained to the patient and the patient is instructed to report any problems."

12. Insertion and removal of the hearing aids: "Patients are instructed on how to insert and remove the hearing aids from their ears and we spend a good portion of time during the delivery process making sure the patient can do this with minimal frustration. The patient is instructed to report problems in the ears if problems should occur."

13. Verification of the hearing aids: "The verification of the fitting is done by running real-ear measurements on all of my patients."

14. Caring for the hearing aids: "All patients are instructed and shown how to clean their hearing aids, insert and remove the batteries, and how to adjust any features and/or controls of the devices. The patient is to report any problems with the fit or the sound quality if anything should arise."

15. Paperwork: "The warranty policy, user manual, and purchase agreement are reviewed with the patient. The follow-up appointments are scheduled as well."

16. "I always call patients the following day to see how they are doing and if they have any questions."

DELIVERY OF A BTE HEARING AID

1. Predelivery of the BTE: Talk out loud, "In our office, we first wash our hands before handling any hearing aid. The earmold and BTE model, size, serial numbers, specifications, battery size, and color are checked against the order form and patient record. A listening check is performed and any needed adjustments are made to the devices prior to delivery. The battery compartment, microphone, receiver, vent, and all movable parts are checked and inspected. I also rub the earmold on my forearm checking to see if there are any sharp edges. I also run a 2-cc coupler measurement to ensure that the hearing aids are up to specifications according to the manufacturer's spec sheet."

2. Listening check: "I always check the contacts of the battery and ensure that the battery fits properly and the door opens and closes with ease. The volume control is checked to make sure you can hear it getting louder and softer and that there is no static or intermittency. Everything appears to be in order."

3. Predelivery adjustments of controls: "The hearing aids are checked against

the patient's audiogram, MCL, and UCL. We make sure that the hearing aid can be read in the manufacturer software and is best-fit accordingly while listening to the hearing aids."

4. Fitting and delivery of the BTE: "I have completed the predelivery inspection, listening check, and adjustments. During the delivery process I go over many points in detail with my patients. We also run real-ear measurements on every patient to help with verification and adjustments of the fitting during the delivery process."

5. Otoscopic inspection: "I perform an otoscopic inspection of the pinna and canal prior to the delivery of the hearing aids."

6. Expectations: "I guide the patient through what to expect and what not to expect from the hearing aids."

7. Family: "I encourage the family to participate in the hearing aid fitting."

8. Introduction: "I wash my hands before starting the fitting and delivery process and clean the earmold as well. I measure and fit the earmold to the BTE. I explain that the earmold fits in the concha and the canal portion of the ear (depending on the earmold model). The hearing aids fit behind the ear. I practice insertion and removal with them."

9. Cleaning: "I instruct patients on the proper cleaning techniques of both the hearing aid and the earmold and have them demonstrate them to me so I can ensure that they understand how to clean the instruments properly."

10. Wearing: "Patients are instructed to wear the hearing aids as much as possible or as much as they feel comfortable. In my office, we give the patient a 2- to 3-week rehabilitation program to follow and regularly scheduled appointments."

11. Feedback: "I explain what feedback is and that the patient may experience feedback or whistling if the earmold tubing is plugged with debris or if it becomes hard over time. Feedback may also occur when the hearing aid microphone is covered."

12. Insertion and removal of the hearing aids: "Patients are instructed on how to insert and remove the earmolds and hearing aids from their ears and we spend a good portion of time during the delivery process making sure the patient can do this with minimal frustration. The patient is instructed to report problems in the ears if problems should occur."

13. Verification of the hearing aids: "The verification of the fitting is done by running real-ear measurements on all of my patients."

14. Caring for the hearing aids: "All patients are instructed and shown how to clean their hearing aids, insert and remove the batteries, and how to adjust any features and/or controls of the devices. The patient is to report any problems with the fit or the sound quality if anything should arise."

15. Paperwork: "The warranty policy, user manual, and the purchase agreement are reviewed with the patient. The follow-up appointments are scheduled as well."

16. "I always call patients the following day to see how they are doing and if they have any questions."

DELIVERY OF AN RIC HEARING AID

1. Predelivery of the RIC: Talk out loud, "In our office, we first wash our hands before handling any hearing aid. The RIC serial numbers, receivers, specifications, battery size, and color are checked against the order form and patient record. A listening check is performed, and any needed adjustments are made to the devices prior to delivery. The battery compartment, microphone, receiver, vent, and all movable parts are checked and inspected. I also run a 2-cc coupler measurement to

ensure that the hearing aids are up to specifications according to the manufacturer's spec sheet."

2. Listening check: "I always check the contacts of the battery and ensure that the battery fits properly, and the door opens and closes with ease. The volume control is checked to make sure you can hear it getting louder and softer and that there is no static or intermittency. Everything appears to be in order."

3. Predelivery adjustments of controls: "The hearing aids are checked against the patient's audiogram, MCL, and UCL. We make sure that the hearing aid can be read in the manufacturer software and is best-fit accordingly while listening to the hearing aids."

4. Fitting and delivery of the RIC: "I have completed the predelivery inspection, listening check, and adjustments. During the delivery process I go over many points in detail with my patients. We also run real-ear measurements on every patient to help with verification and adjustments of the fitting during the delivery process."

5. Otoscopic inspection: "I perform an otoscopic inspection of the pinna and canal prior to the delivery of the hearing aids."

6. Expectations: "I guide the patient through what to expect and what not to expect from the hearing aids."

7. Family: "I encourage the family to participate in the hearing aid fitting."

8. Introduction: "I wash my hands before starting the fitting and delivery process. I explain that the earbud fits in the canal portion of the ear. The hearing aids fit behind the ear. I practice insertion and removal with them."

9. Cleaning: "I instruct patients on the proper cleaning techniques of both the hearing aid and the earbud and have them demonstrate them to me, so I can ensure that they understand how to clean the instruments properly."

10. Wearing: "Patients are instructed to wear the hearing aids as much as possible or as much as they feel comfortable. In my office, we give the patient a 2- to 3-week rehabilitation program to follow and regularly scheduled appointments."

11. Feedback: "I explain what feedback is and that the patient may experience feedback or whistling if the earmold tubing is plugged with debris or if it becomes hard over time. Feedback may also occur when the hearing aid microphone is covered."

12. Insertion and removal of the hearing aids: "Patients are instructed on how to insert and remove the earbuds and hearing aids from their ears and we spend a good portion of time during the delivery process making sure the patient can do this with minimal frustration. The patient is instructed to report problems in the ears if problems should occur."

13. Verification of the hearing aids: "The verification of the fitting is done by running real-ear measurements on all of my patients."

14. Caring for the hearing aids: "All patients are instructed and shown how to clean their hearing aids, insert and remove the batteries, and how to adjust any features and/or controls of the devices. The patient is to report any problems with the fit or the sound quality if anything should arise."

15. Paperwork: "The warranty policy, user manual, and the purchase agreement are reviewed with the patient. The follow-up appointments are scheduled as well."

16. "I always call patients the following day to see how they are doing and if they have any questions."

OTHER RELEVANT INFORMATION

The successful fitting of hearing instruments depends on effectively teaching your patient how to operate and insert the instrument, and many times instructions are not enough. You must guide and counsel the patient and family about what to expect and what *not* to expect from the new instruments. Important terms are:

- *Fitting*—when the patient receives the hearing instrument.
- *Post-fitting*—any visit after the patient is fit with the instrument (any adjustment, verification, or checkup after the initial visit).
- *Fitting verification*—any test, measurement, or exercise you give the patient to verify the success of the fitting.

Fitting, post-fitting, and verification are all critical to successful use. A hearing instrument *does not* restore normal hearing; however, residual hearing is enhanced with the hearing instrument. Show the patient the entire hearing instrument (and earmold). Explain each part, the entire shape, the canal, the outer surface/ faceplate, and the helix, how it sits in or on the ear, and what position it sits in. Demonstrate cleaning the instrument with a soft cloth, the wax pick/loop, and a brush. Teach the patient how to insert and remove the instrument or earmold. Demonstrate the controls on the hearing instrument. Show the patient the battery, the positive side versus the negative side, and how to insert and remove it.

Batteries

The proper handling of batteries is as follows:

- Use only fresh batteries.
- Store batteries in a cool, dry place.
- Do not leave a dead battery in the hearing aid.
- Wipe off the battery if it gets exposed to moisture.
- Do not put batteries in a DRI-AID kit.

- Store batteries separate from medication. Do not put batteries in your mouth or swallow them.
- Give the patient the battery hotline phone number.

BTE and Tubing

- If the instrument is a BTE, it should sit comfortably on the top of the ear and rest along the back of the ear.
- Insert and remove the earmold again.
- Measure the tubing to ensure that overlap of the elbow is 0.125 to 0.25 inch.
- Attach the earmold to the hearing instrument.
- Reinsert the earmold and place the hearing aid behind the ear.
- Check the fit.

Earmolds

Care for earmolds is as follows:

- Keep the earmold free of wax.
- Use the wax loop—never toothpicks!
- Remove moisture bubbles from the tubing. Disconnect the tubing from the BTE and force air through the tube, clearing the moisture. Wait until it is dry and then reconnect it to the BTE.

Changing the Tubing

It is important to change the tubing when the following occurs:

- The tubing starts to harden or deteriorate.
- The tubing separates from either the hearing instrument or the earmold.

- The tubing becomes discolored, twists, splits, or feels too short or too long.
- The earmold hurts, easily becomes dislodged, or does not seat properly in ear, or if feedback occurs for any reason.

Volume Control

Two important points about volume control are as follows:

- Show the patient how to adjust the volume control.
- Normal is a range—*not* an exact spot on the dial!

Telecoil

- Can be automatic when the phone is held up to the hearing aid. ITE and canal instruments may have a switch (like a light switch): M (microphone) and T (telephone) position.

For BTEs:

- Switch from the M (microphone) to the T (telephone) position.
- Turn the volume louder.
- Hold the phone to the hearing instrument.
- Alternate use for assistive listening devices.
- The telecoil can also be automatic when the phone is held up to the hearing aid.

Binaural Amplification

Note the following points with regard to binaural amplification:

- You do not have a poor side.
- You have your sense of direction.
- You wear two instruments quieter than only one.
- Clarity improves.
- You can be "bionic" at will.
- Ease of listening increases.
- MCL: All your conversations with the patient help establish a comfortable listening level.
- UCL: Check uncomfortable levels. Rattle paper, shake keys, and use a noise CD while carrying on a conversation.
- Word discrimination scores: One of the easiest ways to associate an improvement in hearing is with speech discrimination tests. How would you show an improvement?

General Care and Maintenance

The hearing aid must be removed in the following circumstances:

- Washing your hair, face, or shaving
- Under a hair dryer
- Using hair spray
- Showering
- Swimming

Certain Considerations

What might you say about the following?

- Battery door
- Where to store the instruments
- How to clean wax
- General cleaning care
- Dropping the instrument
- In places with high humidity
- Patient troubleshooting
- Changes in hearing or the hearing aid
- Maintenance checkup

Certain Things to Review with the Patient

You should definitely review the following with the patient:

- Always open the battery door at night.
- Do not put your hearing instrument near heat, direct sunlight, or in the glove compartment of your car.
- Remove wax from ITE or canal instruments only with the special tool provided.
- Wipe the instrument with a soft cloth or tissue.
- Protect the instrument from dropping by handling it over a table or sitting on a bed.
- Use a DRI-AID kit or silica gel when moisture or perspiration is a concern.
- Do not attempt to repair the hearing aid.
- Report any change of hearing, hearing instrument function, or ability to handle the instrument.
- Have regular maintenance and checkups every 4 to 6 months.

Paperwork

Regarding paperwork, do the following:

- Fill out guarantees.
- Fill out warranties.
- Review the instruction booklet.
- Review battery size and warnings.
- Fill out and sign the contract.
- Provide copies of these documents to the patient.
- Collect money.
- Make 1-week appointment for follow-up.
- Give the patient the appointment card.
- Give the patient your business card.

Delivery of BTE Hearing Aid

The following is a brief 12-step process for delivering a BTE hearing aid as you would state *out loud* during your examination:

1. "When inserting the earmold, hold on to the outer side near the tubing and gently insert the tip of the earmold at a slight angle into the ear canal."
2. "You can apply slight pressure with your finger on the outside of the earmold to push it into the ear. If needed, you can check the placement in a mirror to ensure that it is properly in place."
3. "Place the hearing instrument behind your ear by lifting it up and over your pinna so that it wraps around your ear."
4. If applicable: "Turn the hearing aid on by setting the MTO switch to the 'M' position and state the 'T' position is used only when using the phone."
5. "Locate the volume control wheel by moving your finger behind your ear. Adjust the volume control. With your fingertip, move the volume wheel in an upward motion, toward the top of your head, and that will increase the volume of the aid."
6. "Turn your hearing aid to the 'O' or off position."
7. "Slide the hearing aid from behind your ear to the front of your ear."
8. "Grab the earmold and gently slide the earmold out of the concha area and slowly turn it toward your nose while pulling it out of your ear canal."
9. "Your hearing aid takes a size 675 [or state whatever the battery size is]."
10. "To insert the battery, remove the colored tab from the battery and pull open the battery door completely."
11. "Insert the battery so that the positive side of the battery that has the plus (+) on its face the same way as the (+) on the battery door, and close the battery door completely."
12. "If you find that you have to force the battery door closed, then you most likely

have the battery in wrong. Remove the battery from the battery door and begin again."

Congratulations, you have now completed the third module! I am hoping that this section was beneficial and helped you to know the flow and process of the fitting and delivery process. This module should serve as a base for what *you* will say and do during this section of the practical exam. I highly recommended that you take what you have learned from this module and write yourself a script ensuring that you have included all the important points. Run through the script once you know how much time you are allotted on your practical exam and be sure to hit on all of it in the time you have. Practice, practice, practice!

MODULE 3 TEST QUESTIONS

1. Which of the following is true about cleaning a hearing instrument?
   a. It is not important
   b. It can be washed with soap and water
   c. It should be cleaned daily
   d. It should be cleaned weekly

2. It is not important perform a predelivery inspection before scheduling your patient to come in for the fitting.
   a. True
   b. False

3. It is important to wash your hands:
   a. Before touching the patient
   b. Before handling the hearing instrument
   c. Before handling the earmold
   d. All of the above

4. It is common practice to verify your fitting using either real-ear measurement, speech mapping, or sound-field measurement.
   a. True
   b. False

5. A vent is:
   a. A hole made in the earmold to hold the tubing
   b. A hole made in the hearing instrument to allow for the passage of air
   c. A hole made in the earmold to allow for the passage of aid
   d. Both B and C

6. Earmold tubing size has an effect on the hearing aid response.
   a. True
   b. False

7. The 3 types of venting that are generally used with earmolds are:
   a. Small, medium, and large
   b. Internal, external, and trench
   c. Diagonal, parallel, and external
   d. None of the above

8. A large vent will effect frequencies between 250 and 1500 Hz.
   a. True
   b. False

9. An open vent earmold will increase the effect on the low frequencies.
   a. True
   b. False

10. Venting is used to:
    a. Improve sound quality
    b. To change the response of the hearing aid
    c. To increase the comfort to the patient
    d. All of the above

11. Having a family member present during the delivery process is an important part of the rehabilitation process.
    a. True
    b. False

12. What is important to perform during your predelivery inspection?
    a. That you received what you ordered
    b. That the hearing aid will read in the manufacturer's software
    c. That the hearing aids works with a battery inserted
    d. All of the above

13. Binaural amplification should always be recommended unless:
    a. You feel the patient cannot afford it
    b. The patient has a unilateral hearing loss
    c. You should never recommend binaural amplification
    d. None of the above

14. It is important to change tubing:
    a. Every year
    b. Every time you see the patient
    c. Never
    d. When the tubing starts to harden

15. Hearing aids should be removed:
    a. Never
    b. When washing your hair
    c. In the car
    d. All of the above

16. Fitting, post-fitting, and verification are all critical to successful use of hearing aids.
    a. True
    b. False

17. It is important to review all of following with the patient except:
    a. What you actually paid for the hearing aid
    b. The battery size and warnings
    c. Warranties
    d. Purchase agreement

18. After the hearing aid delivery, patients should only come back if they are having problems.
    a. True
    b. False

19. A 2-cc coupler measurement should be run on hearing instruments that you just received from the manufacturer.
    a. True
    b. False

20. When performing a listening check, you should always:
    a. Check the telecoil
    b. Insert a battery and open and close the battery door multiple times
    c. Perform it only when the patient is present
    d. Both A and B
    e. All of the above

For more quiz questions for Module 3, visit the companion website and test your knowledge.

MODULE 4

Hearing Instrument Care and Follow-Up

16

Replacing Earmold Tubing

Objectives

- To prepare the candidate to perform the proper procedure for replacing tubing on an earmold

During the practical section of the state exam, most states require candidates to physically replace earmold tubing, not just discuss the steps that one would take to replace the tubing. Make sure you check the material that your state sends prior to the exam so you are aware of what their expectations are when it comes to replacing earmold tubing. States usually provide all of the needed tools and materials for this section of the exam, but for those states that do not provide the necessary tools, ensure that you are familiar with, and have worked with, the tools that they require you to bring. Figure 16–1 shows the more common tools used for replacing earmold tubing, so when preparing for your exam, practice with these tools so that the only thing you need to do is show that you know the proper procedure for replacing the tubing.

Replacing earmold tubing may vary depending on earmold material, acoustic options, and tubing retention. For the purpose of most state exams, states will be testing you on your knowledge about the process and will generally use a hard, lucite-type

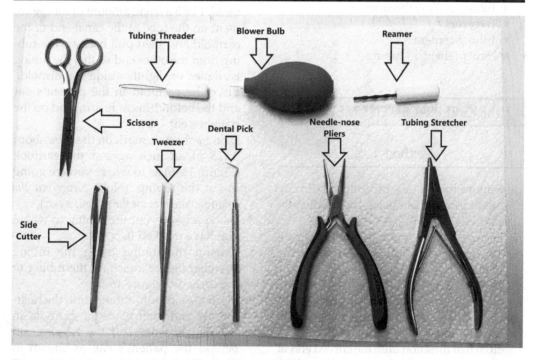

Figure 16–1. Common tools for replacing earmold tubing.

material with a largebore and regularsize tubing, which makes the process easier, since multiple candidates will be changing the tubing on the earmold during the exam.

TOOLS

As previously stated, most states provide the necessary tools for you to use when performing a tubing replacement. It is imperative that you be familiar with, and have handled, all the tools necessary and that you be confident and competent in using them prior to your exam. The following is a list of the tools with which you need to familiarize yourself (see Figure 14–1):

- Dental pick
- Side cutter
- Needlenose pliers
- Tubing stretcher
- Scissors
- Reamer
- Blower bulb
- Tubing puller/threader
- Tweezers
- Tubing cement
- New prebent 13 tubing

TUBING REPLACEMENT METHODS

Method 1

1. Remove the old tube by pulling it directly out of the earmold using the needlenose pliers (Figure 16–2).
2. Ensure that the sound bore is clean, smooth, and free of debris using the reamer and the earmold blower (Figure 16–3).
3. Thread the new tube through the back end of the earmold (the side that faces outside of the body). Once the tubing appears on the other side of the earmold, pull the tube from that direction until the curved end of the tube reaches the outer portion of the

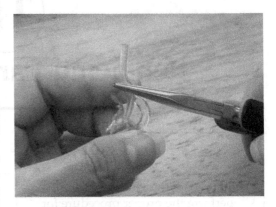

Figure 16–2. Removing old tube with needlenose pliers.

earmold (Figure 16–4A). If you have difficulty threading the tubing through the bore, use the tubing puller/threader to assist you as shown in Figure 16–4B.

4. As shown in Figure 16–5, cut off the excess tubing from the inside portion (canal tip) of the earmold using either a side cutter or scissors. Make sure the tubing is aligned smoothly with the tip of the earmold. Place a small amount of tubing cement on the tube at the canal end of the earmold and then pull back on the tubing from the other end so that the tubing is aligned or slightly inside the earmold.
5. Place the earmold in the patient's ear and the behindtheear hearing aid on the patient's ear.
6. Using a marker, mark on the tube about 0.125 of an inch against the earhook (Figure 16–6) as to where you are going to cut the tubing. (Note: *Never cut the tubing while it is on the patient's ear.*)
7. Using scissors, cut the tubing to where you have marked it.
8. Expand the tubing using the tubing stretcher before attaching the tubing to the earhook (Figure 16–7).
9. Place the earmold tubing onto the hearing aid and then place the earmold in the patient's ear and the hearing aid behind the patient's ear, as shown in Figure 16–8.

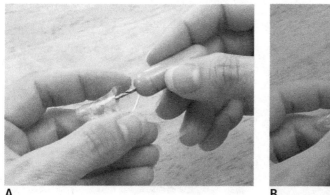 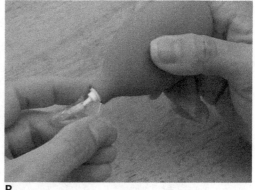

A   B

Figure 16–3. A. A reamer. **B.** An earmold blower bulb.

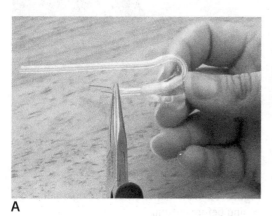 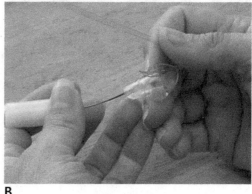

A   B

Figure 16–4. A. Without threader using needle-nose pliers. **B.** With threader.

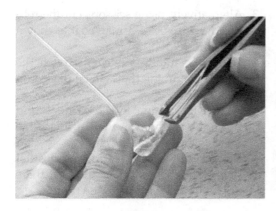 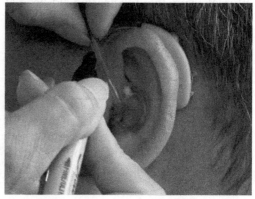

Figure 16–5. Cutting tubing with a side cutter.   **Figure 16–6.** Marking the earmold.

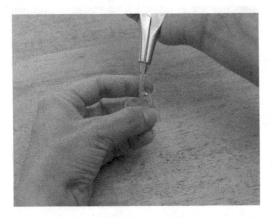

Figure 16–7. A tubing expander.

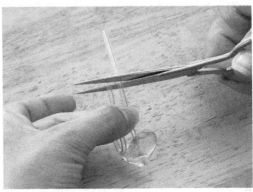

Figure 16–9. Comparison of the old earmold tubing with the new earmold tubing.

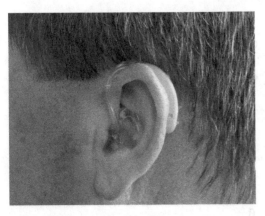

Figure 16–8. Proper placement of earmold and hearing aid on the ear.

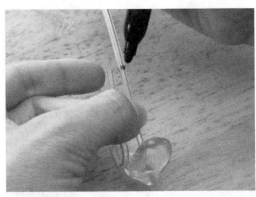

Figure 16–10. Marking new tubing against old tubing before cutting.

10. Make sure that the hearing aid lies flat over the patient's pinna and that there are no kinks or twists in the tubing.

Method 2

1. Follow steps 1 to 4 as shown in method 1.
2. Using the old tube as a comparison, line up the tubes and cut off the excess tubing that attaches to the earhook (Figure 16–9).
3. Alternatively, using scissors, cut the tubing to where you have marked it, as shown in Figure 16–10.
4. Using the tubing stretcher, stretch the end of the tubing that will be placed on the earhook.
5. Attach the tubing to the earhook and place the earmold in the ear. Place the hearing aid behind the ear.
6. Make sure that the hearing aid lies flat over the patient's pinna and that there are no kinks or twists in the tubing.

17

Routine Follow-Up Service

Objectives

- To prepare the candidate to be able to instruct patients in the care and use of their hearing aids
- To prepare the candidate to be able to validate the hearing aid fitting
- To ensure that the candidate has a postfitting process in place for every patient who is fit with hearing aids

Postfitting follow-up care is probably the single most important step in the hearing aid process to determine if the patient will not only use the hearing aids but accept them as well. Postfitting appointments are critical to the success of the hearing aid fitting and include many processes, such as instructions for the patient, counseling, aural rehabilitation, and family involvement.

During your state practical exam, you will most likely need to "pretend" that you are performing a follow-up appointment with a patient, and what you will really be doing is just talking out loud while the proctors assess your knowledge of the important aspect of follow-up patient care and ensure that you have touched on all the important points. So, for the purpose of this manual, we only review the processes and their most basic attributes for when you take your exam, because you will only have a small amount of time to get your points across, not the usual "multiple" office visits that you would have in the real world that entail the actual postfitting care process.

For more in-depth reading on this topic, I have included a list of books in the recommended reading section at the end of this manual. You can also check out the companion website for more information.

POSTFITTING CARE PROCESS

At the initial fitting and delivery of the hearing aids you went over a great deal of information with the patient (review Chapters 13 and 15). For the postfitting process you may want to think about it in terms of a checklist that you will go over at each visit when the patient returns. It is ultimately your responsibility as the hearing health professional to provide this extended care to your patient in order for the fitting to be successful. As you are already aware, there are many factors that go into a successful fitting and it will take time for all of it to fall into place. So, it is extremely important to bring the patient back for routine follow-up appointments (Taylor & Mueller, 2011).

The following is an example of how you can go about your postfitting care. These steps are set up in a way that will help you to remember what the important aspects of this process are. If you already work in a dispensing office and have a postfitting process in place, then use the process with which you are comfortable. If you do not work in a dispensing office or do not have a postfitting process in place, then let this be the foundation for best practice and good habits for you to begin early in your career, a process that will aid in your success and patient satisfaction. Every patient visit should include:

- Questions
- Education
- Communication tips
- Encouragement

One-Week Check

The following is a checklist of what to do at the 1-week check:

- Call the patient the day after delivery to see how she/he is doing.
- Perform an otoscopic inspection on both ears to make sure there are no pressure points caused by the hearing aids and to ensure that the ear canal and tympanic membrane appear healthy.
- Review the wearing schedule "homework" with the patient and discuss her/his responses to your questions and notes that the patient took during that time.
- Do I need to review or finish anything from the initial delivery process that we did not get to during that day?
- Check and review any areas of concern:
  - Tolerance to loud sounds
  - Sharpness or harshness
  - Feedback
  - Occlusion
  - Sound not clear
  - Sound is muffled
  - Sound is tinny
  - Familiar with user controls
  - Telephone use
  - Fit of the instruments
  - Insertion and removal of the instruments
  - TV use
  - Phone use
- Make a list of any actions that you may have taken during this appointment. For example,

programming adjustments or modification to the instruments.
- Make note of any further counseling that you may have provided to the patient and/or family members during this appointment.
- Make note of further recommendations that you made to the patient and provide the patient with the next step of "homework" for the next 1 to 2 weeks.
- Schedule the next appointment.

Two-Week Check

The following is a checklist of what to do at the 2-week check:

- Review concerns and/or problems from the previous appointment.
- Perform an otoscopic inspection on both ears to make sure there are no pressure points caused by the hearing aids and to ensure that the ear canal and tympanic membrane appear healthy.
- Address any new concerns or problems.
- Review the wearing schedule "homework" with the patient and discuss the answers and notes that the patient took during that time.
- Review and encourage family involvement: Keep expectations within realistic bounds for both the patient and family. Provide information to the patient and family. The family needs to:
  - Have reasonable expectations
  - Avoid misconceptions
  - Improve their communication skills
  - Obtain any additional necessary information
  - Learn to soften their voices
- Make a list of any actions that you may have taken during

this appointment—for example, programming adjustments or modification to the instruments.

- Make a note of further recommendations that you made to the patient and provide the patient with the next step of "homework" for the next follow-up appointment.
- Schedule the next appointment for 2 weeks later (or sooner if you are working on continued issues with the patient).

Four-Week Check

- Review concerns and/or problems from the previous appointment.
- Perform an otoscopic inspection on both ears to make sure there are no pressure points caused by the hearing aids and to ensure that the ear canal and tympanic membrane appear healthy.
- Address any new concerns or problems.
- Review the wearing schedule "homework" with the patient and discuss the answers and notes that the patient took during that time.
- Review other ways we can improve communication with hearing aids, such as the following:
  - Use visual cues to increase what we understand correctly.
  - Look at each other when we talk.
  - Provide content and subject matter.
  - Talk slower.
  - Do not yell from another room.
- Review with patients when they should contact you:
  - When there is a change in their hearing
  - If their hearing aid is not working
  - If there have been major changes in their lives concerning:
    - Illness

- Medications
- Weight loss
- Dental work
- General health

- If all is well, then you can discuss the follow-up visit schedule with them (every 3 months):
  - 3-month check
  - 6-month check
  - 9-month check
  - 1-year check

WHAT TO CHECK AT THE APPOINTMENT EVERY 3 MONTHS

Do the following at the appointment every 3 months:

- Review with the patient any problems or concerns that she/he may be experiencing.
- Perform an otoscopic inspection of the patient's ears.
- Perform a thorough cleaning of the instruments to ensure that they are in good working condition.
- Perform a 2-cc coupler measurement to ensure that the hearing aids are up to manufacturer specifications.
- Perform any acoustic adjustments to the instruments, if needed, based on what the patient reports.
- Check the patient's battery supply.
- Ask for referrals.
- Schedule the next 3-month check.

WHAT TO CHECK AT THE YEARLY APPOINTMENT

Do the following at the yearly appointment:

- Review with the patient any problems or concerns that she/he may be experiencing.

- Perform an otoscopic inspection of the patient's ears.
- Perform a thorough cleaning of the instruments to ensure that they are in good working condition.
- Perform a 2-cc coupler measurement to ensure that the hearing aids are up to manufacturer specifications.
- Perform a full audiometric test on the patient to see if there has been any change in hearing.
- Perform any acoustic adjustments to the instruments, if needed, based on what the patient reports or changes in hearing levels

based on your audiometric evaluation.
- Check the patient's battery supply.
- Discuss any hearing aid warranty extensions that may be up at this time and if the patient would like to renew.
- Ask for referrals.
- Schedule the next 3-month check.

REFERENCE

Taylor, B., & Mueller, H. G. (2011). *Fitting and dispensing hearing aids*. San Diego, CA: Plural Publishing.

(18)
Troubleshooting

Objectives

- To provide the candidate with strategies to help identify and alleviate problems with hearing instruments
- To prepare the candidate to know what problems affect the electroacoustic parameters of the hearing instrument
- To teach the candidate to perform a listening check of the hearing instrument
- To teach the candidate how to test the hearing instrument
- To educate the candidate on strategies for correcting problems with the hearing instrument

TROUBLESHOOTING

This chapter focuses on techniques that can be used when troubleshooting patients' complaints about their hearing aids. While we would all like to believe that we have gone through all the initial steps to choose and fit the patient appropriately so that we would not have to fine-tune the hearing aids or physically modify them, the truth is, that is not always the case. Because of this, most state licensing exams focus on the troubleshooting of hearing instruments. Some of the complaints that we discuss may be seen at the initial fitting, whereas others will manifest when the patient comes in for the follow-up appointment. In this chapter we review the most common patient complaints and the steps that one would take to troubleshoot, verify, and correct the problem. We focus on both newer digital hearing aid technology as well as older analog technology so that you understand everything that encompasses a troubleshooting procedure.

For most state exams you will not have to actually perform the task of repairing or correcting the problem that is reported, but you will need to take steps to figure out what could be causing the complaint that is presented and then the steps you would take if you were to correct the problem. Make sure to read the information provided by your state to be sure you know what you are expected to perform during your practical examination. If you are required by your state to bring a hearing aid listener, or if your state supplies one for you, make sure you use it! One of the most important skills that you need to have to be a successful hearing aid dispenser is to be able to listen to the aids and know for what you are listening. Do not assume you know what the problem is based solely on a visual inspection of the hearing aid; you must listen to it. Furthermore, while you are listening to the hearing aid, open and close the battery door, check the taper in the volume control, and check the voltage of the battery if a battery tester is available during the test.

COMMON COMPLAINTS, SYMPTOMS, CAUSES, AND SOLUTIONS

In this section we review the most common complaints and then break them down into what the cause of the complaint could be and then what the solution may be. When presenting the solution, we look at both the physical modifications or repair action(s) that you may have to take as well as acoustic changes that may need to be performed to address the problem.

Complaint of Feedback

Feedback can occur for many different reasons and at any stage along the fitting/ follow-up process. The big key to troubleshooting feedback is asking the patient when the feedback started. If, for instance, it is the initial fit and the patient has yet to wear the instruments, you would most likely approach the feedback troubleshooting differently than you would if the patient has come in for a follow-up appointment and has been wearing the hearing instrument for any length of time. The following is the feedback checklist you would go through for determining the cause of the complaint, followed by the solutions for correcting the problem.

Feedback Checklist

The feedback checklist is as follows:

- Wax in the microphone?
- Wax in the receiver?
- Excessive wax in the ear canal?
- Microphone covered by the ear?
- Earmold/shell too loose?
- Canal length too short?
- Canal length too long and up against the canal wall?
- Excessive jaw movement creating a leak in the seal of the hearing aid?
- Vent too large?
- Volume control turned up too loud or all the way?
- If no volume control, is the gain of the hearing aid close to max for the matrix of the aid?

- Excessive peak in the response curve?

Feedback Solutions

Modification of the Hearing Aid. To modify the hearing aid, take the following relevant action(s):

- Remove the wax from the microphone/receiver.
- Refer patient to have the wax removed from ear.
- Remake the hearing aid (take a new impression).
- Build up the instrument.
- Reduce the vent size.
- Plug the vent.
- Add a damper in the receiver.
- Shorten the canal to prevent the aid from hitting the canal wall.
- Add a canal lock or helix lock.
- Activate the high-frequency potentiometer.

Repair or Programming of the Hearing Aid. To repair or program the hearing aid, take the following relevant action(s):

- Add an extended receiver tube.
- Tighten the fit.
- Lengthen the canal.
- Redirect the receiver.
- Reduce the high-frequency response.
- Add more low-frequency gain.
- Send it to the manufacturer to have the matrix increased.
- Smooth the frequency response of any peaks.

Complaint of Tinniness

This complaint is most often seen when there is an excess of high-frequency gain in the hearing instrument. Patients may describe this as paper rustling, keys rattling, glass, plates, and so forth that are uncomfortable and sharp sounding to them.

Tinniness Solutions

Modification of the Hearing Aid. To modify the hearing aid, take the following relevant action(s):

- Reduce the vent size.
- Add a damper.
- Activate the high-frequency potentiometer.

Repair or Programming of the Hearing Aid. To repair or program the hearing aid, take the following relevant action(s):

- Decrease the slope.
- Reduce the high-frequency gain.
- Add more low-frequency gain.
- Add an extended receiver tube.
- Lengthen the canal of the hearing aid.

Complaint of Occlusion

Patients who are experiencing occlusion may complain that they sound like they are talking in a barrel, that their own voice bothers them, or that they can hear their own breathing or heartbeat. The patient is feeling "plugged up" and it is typically related to the vent size and too much low-frequency amplification.

Occlusion Solutions

Modification of the Hearing Aid. To modify the hearing aid, take the following relevant action(s):

- Shorten the vent.
- Enlarge the vent.
- Bell the canal.
- Taper the canal.
- Shorten the canal.

- Activate the low-frequency potentiometer.

Repair or Programming of the Hearing Aid. To repair or program the hearing aid, take the following relevant action(s):

- Decrease the low-frequency amplification.
- Increase the slope.
- Increase the high-frequency amplification.
- If it is a fit issue and the ear is too small to accommodate a larger vent, then consider changing to a different model which would allow for larger venting.

Complaint of Weak Performance

When patients come in with the complaint of the hearing aid being "weak," there are a few different culprits that could cause this type of complaint. So as with troubleshooting feedback, there is a checklist that should be completed to narrow down what the cause could be.

Weak-Performance Checklist

The weak-performance checklist is as follows:

- Wax or debris in the receiver or receiver protection?
- Wax or debris in the receiver tube?
- Wax or debris in the microphone or microphone cover?
- Debris on the battery contacts?
- Weak or bad battery?
- Low-voltage batteries?
- Inappropriate matrix for the hearing loss?
- Inappropriate programming for the hearing loss?
- Decrease in hearing?
- Receiver tube pushed up against the canal wall blocking the sound?

Weak-Performance Solutions

Modification of the Hearing Aid. To modify the hearing aid, take the following relevant action(s):

- Clean the wax or debris from the receiver.
- Clean the wax or debris from the microphone.
- Clean the battery contacts.
- Perform a listening check with a new battery.

Repair or Programming of the Hearing Aid. To repair or program the hearing aid, take the following relevant action(s):

- Run a 2-cc coupler measurement on the instrument to see if it is up to ANSI specification (ANSI, 2003).
- If there is no change in hearing and the aid is up to specification, increase gain and/or output.
- If the hearing loss has changed, reprogram appropriately.
- If the aid is not up to specification, send it to the manufacturer for repair.
- If the aid is pulled out slightly from the patient's ear and the patient reports the aid to be louder and clearer, then the canal direction is probably off. If there is an extended receiver tube, try cutting it and inserting the aid back into the patient's ear and see if that helps. If it does not help, then a remake of the aid would be needed by the manufacturer to correct the canal direction.

Complaint of Intermittency or Fading

The complaint of fading is usually described as the hearing instrument gradually going down in volume and then gradually coming back up to normal, whereas the intermittent complaint is described as the hearing aid going dead for a period of time and then starting to work again over a period of time.

Solutions for Intermittency or Fading

Modification of the Hearing Aid. To modify the hearing aid, take the following relevant action(s):

- Clean any wax or debris that may be in the receiver.
- Clean any wax or debris that may be in the receiver tubing.

Repair or Programming of the Hearing Aid. To repair or program the hearing aid, take the following relevant action(s):

- Send it to the manufacturer to check for a loose wire.
- Address any issues with the circuit.
- Change the matrix.
- Depending on fitting software with digital hearing aids, consult the manufacturer for features or programming adjustments to make.
- If the hearing aid cuts off with jaw movement, remake it and redirect the receiver.

Complaint of Dead Hearing Aid

When patients complain of the hearing instrument being dead, generally they mean just that: the hearing aid is not amplifying at all. Follow the checklist to troubleshoot this complaint.

Dead Hearing Aid Checklist

The dead hearing aid checklist is as follows:

- Is the battery dead?
- Is the receiver plugged?

- Is the microphone plugged?
- Is the battery not making contact?
- Is the battery inserted properly?
- Is it the correct-size battery?
- Are there wires in the way when you close the battery door?

Solutions for Dead Hearing Aid

Modification of the Hearing Aid.

- Check the hearing aid with a new battery.
- Clean the receiver.
- Clean the microphone.
- Adjust and pull down on the battery contacts.

Repair of the Hearing Aid. To repair the hearing aid, send it to the manufacturer for repair.

Complaint of Excessive Battery Drain

Patients may complain that they are not getting the specified hours from their hearing aid batteries, that their batteries are not lasting as long, or that they are going through more batteries than with their previous hearing aids. Make sure you ask the patient how long the batteries are lasting and see if it is anywhere close to where it should be. We refer to battery drain in terms of the measure of milliamperes; each battery has a milliampere rating and it is listed as mAh, or milliamps per hour. To determine battery drain, you would divide the milliamp rating by the drain figure:

Battery life = battery rating (mAh) / battery current drain

For example, if a battery has a rating of 300 mAh and the hearing aid requires 3 mA of battery current, then the battery life would be 100 hr.

Battery-Drain Checklist

The battery-drain checklist is as follows:

- Is the patient turning the hearing aid off at night or when it is not in use?
- Is the patient opening the battery door at night or when it is not in use?
- Is the patient using recycled batteries?
- Are the batteries fresh?
- Are the battery contacts clean?
- Is the patient in a lot of noise to where the hearing aid could be in compression a majority of the time, taxing the circuit and causing greater battery drain?

Solutions for Battery Drain

Modification of the Hearing Aid. To modify the hearing aid, take the following relevant action(s):

- Measure the hearing aid on a battery-drain meter.
- Have the patient keep a journal of his/her battery use.

Repair of the Hearing Aid. To repair the hearing aid, take the following relevant action(s):

- Decrease the hearing aid matrix, as the higher the gain and output of a hearing aid, the greater the battery drain.
- Send it in for repair.

Complaint of Noisy or Distorted Hearing Aid

This complaint may be caused by circuit noise or microphone noise and should not be confused with the complaint of background noise that we discuss next.

Solutions for Noisy or Distorted Hearing Aid

Testing of the Hearing Aid. To test the hearing aid, run it in a test box and determine whether or not it has high distortion.

Repair of the Hearing Aid. To repair the hearing aid, send it to the manufacturer for repair.

Complaint of Background Noise

When a patient complains of noise, make sure you ask the patient to describe it to you as accurately as possible. You need to be able to determine if the noise is related to the hearing aid and circuit or to low-frequency amplification.

Background-Noise Checklist

The background-noise checklist is as follows:

- What type of noise is it?
- Is it steady state?

- Is it intermittent?
- Is it the "noise" of normal environmental sounds?
- Is it wind?
- What is the patient's reaction to the noise?

Solutions for Background Noise

Modification of the Hearing Aid. To modify the hearing aid, take the following relevant action(s):

Activate the low-frequency potentiometer or low-cut switch.

- Decrease the low-frequency amplification (with programmable hearing aids).
- Decrease/shorten the vent.

REFERENCE

American National Standards Institute (ANSI). (2003). *American National Standard for specification of hearing aid characteristics.* ANSI S3.22–2003. New York, NY: Author.

MODULE 4

Putting It All Together

There is a hands-on section on almost all state examinations for earmold tubing replacement, patient follow-up care, and troubleshooting various hearing aids. The way each state tests this section may vary to some degree, so you must read *all* of the information provided to you by your state to know what is expected of you. What does remain fairly consistent is the way in which *you* go about these processes, so that is what is presented here.

RETUBING THE EARMOLD

To retube the earmold, do the following:

1. Before tubing an earmold, you must always wash your hands.
2. Make sure that the area that you will be working on is clean and sanitary.
3. Use a clean white towel on which to place all of your cleaned and sanitized materials and tools.
4. Remove the old tube from the earmold and then clean the earmold with alcohol.
5. The new tube is placed through the earmold and angled to the right or left so it can fit comfortably over the pinna and connect with the BTE hearing aid ear hook. A small amount of glue can be used to help hold the tube in place in the earmold. (See Chapter 16 for the step-by-step process for replacing earmold tubing.)
6. The BTE is then cleaned and checked, volume control wheels, MTO switches, memory buttons, and so forth should be checked and be in good working condition.
7. The earmold is then placed in the patient's ear and the BTE is placed behind the pinna.
8. The tubing is then marked with a marker to where you will need to cut for a proper fit of the tube on the ear-hook.
9. The earmold and BTE is then removed from the patient's ear and the tubing is then cut to where you have marked it on the tube. (Note: *Never* cut the tubing while it is in the patient's ear.) Attach the earmold to the BTE and then place it on the patient's ear.
10. Wash your hands when you are finished.

ASSESSING THE BTE, RIC, OR ITE

To assess the BTE or ITE, do the following:

1. Before beginning, we always wash our hands.
2. Ensure that the area that you will be working on is clean and sanitary.
3. Use a clean white towel on which to put all of your cleaned and sanitized tools and materials.
4. The hearing aid should be handled with a tissue or sanitary cloth.
5. The shell or case of the hearing aid is cleaned.
6. Patients are then asked what specific problems they are having.
7. Ask them about the fit, battery, cleaning, and wearing time.
8. Inspect the patient's ear canals to look for any wax or debris that may be causing a problem such as blocking of the ear canal.
9. The ITE is physically inspected.
10. Visually check the shell, receiver tubing, volume control wheel, memory

button, and then open and close the battery door.

11. With an otoscope, check the receiver, vent, and microphone.
12. For a BTE, follow the same steps as above but also ensure that you remove the ear-hook to see if it is blocked.
13. Also remove the earmold from the ear-hook and check the tubing and earmold as well.
14. For an RIC device, remove the earbud and check the wax filter.
15. On all devices, perform a listening check while checking the volume control or memory buttons to make sure they are in good working condition.
16. Clean the hearing aid once again before returning it to the patient.
17. Wash your hands when finished.

TROUBLESHOOTING HEARING AID COMPLAINTS AND PROBLEMS

Follow the steps below to troubleshoot:

1. Wash your hands before handling the hearing aid.
2. Handle the hearing aid with a tissue or sanitary cloth.
3. Test the hearing aid battery and visually inspect the battery contacts in the hearing aid.
4. Check the microphone and receiver for any debris or blockage using an otoscope (if available).
5. Visually check the microphone with an otoscope (if available) to see if it has been pushed in or damaged.
6. Check the volume control, memory button, and any other switches while performing a listening check to ensure that they are functioning properly.
7. If the complaint is that the hearing aid feeds back or whistles, state that you would check the patient's ear canal to

make sure they are clear and free of wax and debris.

8. If the complaint is that the hearing aid is dead or weak, check the battery on the battery tester to make sure that it is a good battery.
9. If the battery is weak or dead, state that you would change the battery with a new battery.
10. If the complaint is of a hollow, nasal, echoing, or tinny sound, the potentiometers and vent should be checked to make sure they are properly adjusted.
11. If the complaint is static, the volume control and the battery contacts should be checked and then state that a repair may be needed.
12. If the complaint is that the aid is too loud, the hearing aid should be checked, and 2-cc coupler measurements should be run on the aid to make sure it is up to specifications and appropriate for the hearing loss by comparing it with the patient's audiogram, MCL, UCL, and the spec sheet provided by the manufacturer.
13. After troubleshooting each instrument, wash your hands.

OTHER POSSIBLE HANDS-ON PROCEDURES

There are other possible procedures that you may be asked to perform during your state practical exam. I cannot stress enough how important it is to read *all* of the information provided to you by your state to know what is expected of you! Ensure that you are comfortable with all aspects of the hands-on sections and that you have practiced and then practiced again, so that when it comes time for your exam, you are experienced and proficient in all aspects of hearing aid dispensing.

Congratulations, you have completed the fourth and final module of this manual!

MODULE 4 TEST QUESTIONS

1. Which of the following is not part of the postfitting visit?
   a. Education
   b. Tympanometry
   c. Communication Tips
   d. Encouragement

2. It is fine to cut the tubing while the earmold is in the patient's ear.
   a. True
   b. False

3. It is important to wash your hands:
   a. Before assessing a hearing aid
   b. Before performing otoscopic inspection
   c. Before handling the earmold
   d. All of the above

4. It is important to call your patient to check in the day after delivery.
   a. True
   b. False

5. What is the first thing you should check for if a patient complains that his hearing aid is dead?
   a. The microphone
   b. The receiver
   c. The tubing
   d. The battery

6. You should always perform an otoscopic exam on your patient when troubleshooting their hearing aids.
   a. True
   b. False

7. Why should a 2-cc coupler measurement be run on hearing aids?
   a. To see if they are amplifying
   b. To see if they are dead
   c. To see if they are up to ANSI specs
   d. None of the above

8. Which of the following is not a solution for occlusion?
   a. Enlarge the vent
   b. Close the vent
   c. Adjust low frequency gain
   d. Taper canal

9. The complaint of tinniness is often seen when there are is an excess of high frequency gain.
   a. True
   b. False

10. At a yearly appointment you should not:
    a. Perform an otoscopic inspection of the patient's ears
    b. Perform a full audiometric evaluation
    c. Make acoustic adjustments to the instruments as needed
    d. Try and sell the patient new hearing aids

11. You should only ask for referrals if you know your patient well and are comfortable asking them.
    a. True
    b. False

12. What is important to perform during your predelivery inspection?
    a. That you received what you ordered
    b. That the hearing aid will read in the manufacturer's software
    c. That the hearing aids works with a battery inserted
    d. All of the above

13. Binaural amplification should always be recommended unless:
    a. You feel the patient cannot afford it
    b. The patient has a unilateral hearing loss
    c. You should never recommend binaural amplification
    d. None of the above

14. It is important to change tubing:
    a. Every year
    b. Every time you see the patient
    c. Never
    d. When the tubing starts to harden

15. Hearing aids should be removed:
    a. Never
    b. When washing your hair

c. In the car
d. All of the above

For more quiz questions for Module 4, visit the companion website and test your knowledge.

Glossary

A

Abbreviated Profile of Hearing Aid Benefit (APHAB): a self-assessment inventory that patients take and report the amount of trouble they are having in various environments when it comes to communication and noise.

Acoustic feedback: a whistle caused by the recirculation of the acoustic output leaving the receiver of a hearing aid back into the microphone.

Acoustic gain: the difference in decibels between the intensity or loudness of the input signal and the intensity or loudness of the output signal of a hearing aid.

Acoustic impedance: the total opposition to the flow of acoustic energy to the middle ear.

Acoustic neuroma: a tumor of the auditory nerve (8th cranial nerve) involving the nerve sheath.

Acoustic output: the output of a hearing aid which equals the input plus the gain $(I+G=O)$.

Acoustic trauma: sudden exposure to a loud sound traumatizing the inner ear and causing permanent damage.

Acquired hearing loss: a hearing loss that has an onset after birth, which can occur any time in one's life.

Admittance: the opposite of impedance; measure of how much energy flows through the system.

Air–bone gap (ABG): the amount in decibels by which the air-conduction threshold differs from the bone-conduction threshold and any frequency.

Air conduction (AC): the transmission of sound waves to the inner ear by way of the outer and middle ear.

Amplifier: an electronic sound processor located inside of a hearing aid that increases the incoming signal to improve the audibility of the outgoing signal.

American National Standards Institute (ANSI): an organization that oversees the creation and use of guidelines that impact the profession of hearing aid dispensing. The guideline includes but is not limited to audiometer, hearing aid specifications, speech mapping, etc.

Analog hearing aid: system of amplification where the electrical signal is analogous to the acoustical input signal in intensity, frequency, and temporal patterns.

Anotia: absence of a pinna.

Aseptic technique: a procedure to be performed under sterile conditions.

Assistive listening devices (ALDs): adjunct hearing devices used to improve signal-to-noise ratio for communication and the performance of activities in specific environments. ALDs include devices such as telephone amplifiers, infrared and FM personal amplifiers, and closed captioning equipment for television use.

Asymmetrical hearing loss: the characteristics of degree and configuration of the loss are different between ears.

Atresia: the complete closure of the external auditory canal.

Attenuation: the reduction of energy, i.e., sound.

Audiogram: a graph that represents the results of a hearing test showing hearing threshold as a function of frequency.

Audiometer: an instrument used for measuring hearing thresholds using both air and bone conduction methods.

Audiometry: also known as an audiometric evaluation; a procedure that measures a person's hearing sensitivity by way of an audiometer, relative to the sensitivity of average hearing.

Auditory nerve: also known as the acoustic nerve; it is the VIIIth cranial nerve, which connects the inner ear to the brain and comprises both the auditory and vestibular branches.

Auditory perception: ability to interpret, identify, and attach meaning to sound.

Aural rehabilitation: the treatment and training of those who acquired hearing loss after language development to improve communication skills.

Auricle: also known as the pinna; it is the outer cartilaginous part of the ear that is responsible for localization and collecting sound.

Autocoil: also known as an automatic telecoil (see telecoil).

B

Barotrauma: damage to the middle ear caused by a rapid change of pressure.

Battery: the power supply for a hearing aid.

Behind-the-ear hearing aid (BTE): a style of hearing aid in which the electronic portion of the hearing aid (including battery, microphone, speaker, amplifier, etc.) is located on top of or behind the ear. The electronic portion is connected via a piece of tubing to an earmold, which is in the ear.

BiCROS hearing aid: bilateral contralateral routing of signal; this type of system is used when there is one dead ear and one ear with hearing loss that can be fit with amplification. There is a microphone on both sides of the head that delivers the signal from the unaidable ear to the aidable ear.

Bilateral hearing loss: loss of hearing in both ears.

Binaural: pertaining to both sides or both ears.

Bing test: a tuning fork test that utilizes the occlusion effect. It tests for the presence or absence of a conductive hearing loss.

Bone conduction: the process by which sound travels to the inner ear and brain by way of the mastoid process, bypassing the outer and middle ear.

Bone conduction threshold: the lowest level in which a person can hear 50% of the time by presenting a tone using a bone oscillator on the mastoid bone.

Bridge-and-brace technique: a safety technique for holding equipment when used on a patient. Both hands need to be touching and act as one, as the equipment being used rests somewhere on the two hands. When approaching the patient, both hands and the equipment act as one as you rest your hands firmly on the patient's head. This prevents harm to the patient if the patient moves her/his head.

Broadband noise: a sound containing a wide range of frequencies.

C

Cerumen: also known as earwax; it is a secretion from ceruminous glands of the external ear canal that keeps it protected from foreign bodies.

Cholesteatoma: a tumor that occurs in the middle ear and mastoid air cell system that is an abnormal accumulation of fats and epithelium from outside the middle ear.

Cleaning: the process of removing debris, decreasing the number of microorganisms that are present.

Cochlea: snail-shaped structure in the inner ear that contains receptor organs essential to hearing.

Cochlear implant: a medical prosthetic device that is surgically placed in the mastoid and the inner ear. It contains a coil and a series of electrodes that bypasses damaged structures in the inner ear and indirectly stimulates the auditory nerve. The purpose is to provide sound to patients with profound hearing loss.

Completely-in-the-canal hearing aid, a.k.a. CIC hearing aid: a hearing aid that is designed so that most of the electronics are located in the ear canal. The smallest style of hearing aid currently available.

Compliance: the opposite of stiffness.

Conductive hearing loss: a loss that occurs when sound is not transmitted efficiently through the outer and middle ear.

Configuration of hearing loss: the shape of a hearing loss; a way to describe the way an audiogram looks.

Congenital: to be born with.

Congenital hearing loss: the presence of hearing loss at or before birth.

Corner audiogram: an audiogram configuration in which there is a severe to profound loss in the low frequencies, no response in the mid or high frequencies.

CROS hearing aid: contralateral routing of signals; this type of system is used when there is one dead ear and one normal hearing ear that does not require amplification. There is a microphone on both sides of the head which delivers the signal from the dead ear to the normal ear. The device on the normal ear also has a receiver to accept the signal from the dead ear.

Cross-contamination: the passing of bacteria, microorganisms, or other harmful substances indirectly from one patient to another through improper or unsterile procedures, equipment, hearing aids, or earmolds.

D

Damping: the decrease in amplitude of the acoustic signal across the frequency range (can be accomplished by using filters, lamb's wool, or dampers).

Decibel (dB): the unit used to measure the intensity or loudness of sound.

Degree of hearing loss: the severity of a hearing loss.

Dermatitis: see eczema.

Disinfecting: the process of killing most germs by using a disinfectant by either spraying it on the surface or by immersing it.

Dynamic range: the difference between the speech reception threshold (SRT) and the uncomfortable loudness level (UCL) for speech.

E

Ear canal: also known as the external auditory meatus and external auditory canal.

The air-filled canal on the side of the head that begins at the concha of the pinna to the eardrum (tympanic membrane).

Eardrum: also known as the tympanic membrane. A thin layer of skin that separates the ear canal from the middle ear cavity. The eardrum converts sound waves into vibrations.

Ear-hook: part of a behind-the-ear hearing aid that is designed to bend over the top of the ear and connect the hearing aid to the tubing of the earmold.

Earmold: a custom-made earpiece that fits in the external canal to conduct amplified sound from the receiver of the hearing aid to the tympanic membrane.

Effective masking (EM): the minimal amount of masking noise that is required to just mask out a signal.

Etiology: in reference to hearing, it is the source or cause of a hearing loss.

Eustachian tube: the channel connecting the throat and the middle ear cavity which is utilized to equalize the pressure in the middle ear cavity to the pressure in the atmosphere surrounding the body.

Exostosis: a bony growth in the ear canal that is generally covered in cartilage.

External auditory canal: (see ear canal)

External ear: the outside portion of the auditory system comprising the pinna and external auditory canal.

External otitis: an infection that forms in the skin of the external auditory canal that is frequently seen in swimmers and people who have water trapped in the ear canal.

F

Feedback: an unwanted high-pitched whistling or squealing sound due to output sound leaking from the hearing aid. The hearing aid's microphone picks up its own output and reamplifies it.

Flat audiogram: a description of the audiogram when the thresholds vary between 10 and 15 dB at all frequencies.

Fluctuating hearing loss: hearing loss that is always changing over time.

Footplate: portion of the stapes bone that is attached to the oval window.

Frequency: in acoustics it is the number of cycles per second or hertz; the number of vibrations occurring during a second, resulting in the perceived pitch of a sound. For example, the more cycles per second, the higher the pitch of the sound.

Functional gain: the difference in decibels between the aided and unaided thresholds of hearing.

Functional hearing loss: also known as non-organic hearing loss. It is the exaggeration of the severity of thresholds.

G

Gain: the difference between the input at the microphone of a hearing aid and the output at the receiver of a hearing aid (I−O=G). It is the amount of amplification a hearing aid can provide.

Gently sloping audiogram: an audiogram configuration with a gradual reduction from lower to high frequencies.

H

Hair cells: sensory cells of the inner ear, which are topped with hair-like structures (stereocilia), which transform the mechanical energy of sound waves by a bending or shearing motion within the organ of Corti.

Hard of hearing: a term used to describe an individual whose sense of hearing is significantly impaired.

Hearing aid: a miniature amplifier that is designed to bring amplified sound to the ear by changing acoustic energy into an electrical signal back to an acoustic signal. A hearing aid consists of a microphone, amplifier, and receiver.

Hearing aid dispenser: also known as a hearing instrument specialist; a person licensed by a state to dispense hearing aids.

Hearing level (HL): the threshold in reference to audiometric zero.

Hearing loss: refers to the partial or total inability to hear sounds in one or both ears.

Hertz: cycles per second.

Hyperacusis: a sensitivity to loud sounds.

I

Idiopathic: occurring without known cause.

Immittance: a term used to describe the measurements of impedance and admittance.

Impedance: see acoustic impedance.

Impression: a cast or mold of the external ear that is used to make an earmold or custom hearing aid.

Incus: also known as anvil; the middle bone of the ossicular chain.

Induction coil: also know as telecoms and/or autocoil; a part inside of a hearing aid that is activated by electromagnetic current flow coming from a telephone or assistive listening device.

Infectious disease: a disease caused by the entrance into the body of organisms (as bacteria, protozoans, fungi, or viruses) which grow and multiply there.

Inner ear: part of the ear that is buried in the skull that contains both the organ of hearing (the cochlea) and the organ of balance (the labyrinth). It converts mechanical energy to electrochemical energy.

Input: the incoming signal to the microphone of a hearing aid.

Interaural attenuation: is the loss of acoustic (sound) energy of a sound as it travels from the test ear across the head to the opposite ear.

In-the-canal (ITC) hearing aid: a style of hearing aid that is smaller than an ITE hearing aid, it usually fills up a portion of the ear canal and a small portion of the outer ear.

In-the-ear (ITE) hearing aid: a style of hearing aid in which all the parts of the hearing aid are fit into the concha or bowl area of the pinna and the ear canal.

L

Labyrinth: a system of interconnecting pathways in the inner ear. The labyrinth consists of the bony portion that contains perilymph and the membranous portion that contains endolymph.

Labyrinthitis: a viral or bacterial infection or inflammation of the inner ear.

Listening stethoscope: a device used to listen to a hearing aid for the purpose of assessing the hearing aid's performance.

Localization: the ability to determine where sound is coming from.

M

Malingering: the act of deliberately exaggerating a hearing loss.

Malleus: also known as the hammer; it is the first and largest of the bones of the ossicular chain, which is connected to the tympanic membrane.

Masking: the process by which a noise is introduced to the nontest ear to prevent that ear from responding when testing the opposite ear.

Masking noise: a sound that is introduced into an ear for the purpose of covering up an unwanted sound or to keep the nontest ear busy during audiometric testing.

Mastoid process: the protrusion of the temporal bone behind the ear.

Mastoidectomy: Surgical procedure to remove infected cells from the mastoid bone.

Ménière's disease: an inner ear disorder that is caused by an excess of endolymph fluid and is often accompanied by symptoms such as fluctuating hearing loss, dizziness, and tinnitus.

Microphone: the part of the hearing aid that converts acoustic energy to electrical energy; input transducer.

Microtia: a very tiny external auditory canal that is congenital in nature.

Middle ear: the air-filled cavity that contains the ossicular chain, which begins at the tympanic membrane and ends at the oval window that leads to the inner ear.

Mixed hearing loss: a hearing loss that has both conductive and sensorineural components.

Monaural: pertaining to one side or one ear.

Monitored live voice (MLV): the presentation of a live speech signal through a microphone on the audiometer. The voice is monitored by a VU meter on the audiometer.

Most comfortable loudness (MCL): the level which a listener designates as the most comfortable level to listen to for speech or tones.

N

Noise–induced hearing loss: a hearing loss caused by exposure to very loud sounds.

Noise-notch: a common audiogram configuration for people with hearing loss due to noise exposure. The notch is generally seen as a sensorineural hearing loss with maximum hearing loss typically between 3000 and 6000 Hz.

Nonorganic hearing loss: see functional hearing loss.

Nontest ear (NTE): the ear that we want to "keep busy" with the masking noise.

O

Occluded: to be obstructed or closed off.

Occlusion effect (OE): the enhancement of bone conduction thresholds at 1000 Hz and below when the ears become occluded.

Ossicles: the chain of the three bones—malleus, incus, and stapes—in the middle ear that form the ossicular chain.

Ossicular discontinuity: when the bones of the middle ear become altered, causing them to not function properly together.

Ossicular fixation: when the bones of the middle ear become ossified and unable to move.

Otalgia: pain in the ear.

Otitis: inflammation of the ear.

Otitis externa: an inflammation of the skin of the outer ear and/or external auditory canal that is caused by an infection.

Otitis media: any infection of the middle ear.

Otorrhea: any discharge from the outer or middle ear.

Otosclerosis: a bony growth in the middle ear that usually occurs around the footplate of the stapes, causing the stapes to remain fixed and unable to move.

Otoscope: an instrument used to visually examine the external auditory canal and the tympanic membrane.

Otoscopy: the process of examining the external ear canal and the tympanic membrane with an otoscope.

Ototoxicity: a hearing loss that occurs by taking drugs that are poisonous to the ear.

Outer ear: the external portion of the ear consisting of the auricle and the ear canal.

Output: see acoustic output.

Overmasking: when there is too much masking present to effectively mask; when each 10 dB increase in masking shifts the hearing threshold by 10 dB or more above the plateau.

P

Perforation: a hole in tissue or an organ. Most commonly seen in the tympanic membrane.

Phonetically balanced words: a list of monosyllabic words that are used to determine a person's speech discrimination score (SDS).

Pinna: part of the outer ear, also known as the auricle.

Plateau: the point in masking when the level of masking noise can be raised or lowered by 15 dB in the nontest ear without affecting the threshold of the test ear.

Polyps: growths in the external auditory canal.

Postauricular: behind the ear.

Presbycusis: age-related hearing loss.

Progressive hearing loss: loss of hearing that presents slowly over time.

Pure tone: a tone that occurs at only one frequency.

Pure-tone average (PTA): the average of thresholds in each ear at three frequencies: 500, 1000, and 2000 Hz.

R

Real-ear measurement: the measurement of a human subject's ear, not an artificial ear.

Receiver: the part of the hearing aid that converts the amplified electrical signal back to an acoustic signal.

Recruitment: a phenomenon in which the person perceives an abnormal increase in loudness with minimal increase in intensity.

Reliability: when you can repeat a test and get the same results every time.

Retrocochlear: everything after the cochlea, that is, auditory nerve and brain.

Rising or reverse slope hearing loss: a configuration of hearing loss that is greater in the low frequencies and better hearing in the high frequencies.

Round window: the membrane that separates the middle ear from the inner ear.

S

Schwartz's sign: noted in some cases of otosclerosis, it is a pinkish or reddish glow that can be seen through the tympanic membrane.

Sensorineural hearing loss: hearing loss caused when there is damage to the inner ear (cochlea) or to the nerve pathways from the inner ear to the brain.

Shadow or mirror audiogram: a configuration of an audiogram when one ear "mirrors" the other because the tone has become loud enough and crosses over for the better ear to hear.

Ski-slope audiogram: also called a high frequency hearing loss or precipitous loss; hearing is better in the low frequencies and then severely drops in the high frequencies.

Sound bore: the hole made in the earmold that holds the tubing and allows for the passage of amplified sound into the ear.

Speech audiometry: the portion of an audiological evaluation that uses speech stimuli to measure the auditory system.

Speech discrimination score (SDS): also known as speech recognition score or word recognition score; the percentage of phonetically balanced words that an individual repeats correctly when presented at a comfortable listening level.

Speech reception threshold (SRT): the lowest level an individual can understand 50% of the time based on a list of spondee words.

Spondee word: a word that consists of two syllables presented with equal stress.

Stable hearing loss: no change in hearing over time.

Standard precautions: a set of infection control practices used to prevent transmission of diseases that can be acquired by contact with blood, body fluids, nonintact skin (including rashes), and mucous membranes.

Stapedectomy: an operation that is used in those with otosclerosis, in which the stapes is removed and a prosthetic is put in its place.

Stapes: also known as the stirrup; it the third and smallest of the bones in the middle ear and connects to the oval window.

Stenosis: narrowing of the external auditory canal.

Sterilizing: the process of removing 100% of the microorganisms and their spores so that they cannot reproduce.

Sudden hearing loss: loss of hearing that occurs quickly.

Symmetrical hearing loss: the characteristics of degree and configuration of the loss are the same in both ears.

T

Telecoil: also known as a T-coil; it is an induction coil built into hearing aids that pick up electromagnetic signals.

Test ear (TE): the ear for which we want to obtain the threshold.

Threshold: the lowest level of a signal (tone or speech) that a person can hear 50% of the time.

Tinnitus: the sensation of any sound, such as ringing, roaring, hissing, or buzzing in the ears or head.

Tympanic membrane (TM): see eardrum.

Tympanogram: a graphic representation of the air pressure and compliance of the middle ear.

Tympanometry: measures how much sound bounces back off the TM as air pressure changes in the outer ear.

U

Uncomfortable loudness level (UCL): the level at which a tone or speech becomes intolerable for an individual. Also known as the threshold of discomfort (TD) or the loudness discomfort level (LDL).

Undermasking: occurs when the masking noise presented to the better ear is not loud enough to eliminate crossover and occurs more commonly in air conduction testing.

Unilateral: one ear.

Unilateral hearing loss: loss of hearing in only one ear.

V

Vent: the hole made in the earmold that allows for passage of air and sound to reach the tympanic membrane.

Abbreviations

ABG air–bone gap
AC air conduction
AD right ear
AGC automatic gain control
AI articulation index
ALD assistive listening device
ANL acceptable noise level
ANSI American National Standards Institute
APHAB Abbreviated Profile of Hearing Aid Benefit
AR aural rehabilitation
AS left ear
AU both ears

BC bone conduction
BiCROS bilateral contralateral routing of signals
BTE behind the ear

CDC Centers for Disease Control and Prevention
CIC completely in the canal
COAT characteristics of amplification tool
COSI Client Oriented Scale of Improvement

daPa decapascals
dB decibels
DNR digital noise reduction
DNT did not test
DSP digital signal processing

EAC external auditory canal
EM earmold/effective masking
ENT ear, nose, and throat

FDA Food and Drug Administration
F/U follow-up

HAE hearing aid evaluation
HFHL high-frequency hearing loss
HHIA Hearing Handicap Inventory for Adults

HHIE Hearing Handicap Inventory for the Elderly
HL hearing loss/hearing level
Hx history
Hz hertz

IA interaural attenuation
IHC inner hair cell
IROS ipsilateral routing of signal
ITC in the canal
ITE in the ear

LDL loudness discomfort level
LE left ear

MCL most comfortable loudness
MLV monitored live voice
mmho millimhos
MPO maximum power output

NAL National Acoustic Laboratories
NAEL National Association of Earmold Labs
NFMI near-field magnetic induction
NIHL noise-induced hearing loss
NTE nontest ear
NU 6 Northwestern University List #6

OC open canal
OE occlusion effect
OHC outer hair cells
OHSAH Occupational Health and Safety Agency for Healthcare
OM otitis media
OSHA Occupational Safety and Health Administration
OSPL output sound pressure level

PB phonetically balanced
PTA pure-tone average

RE right ear
REAG real-ear aided gain
REAR real-ear aided response

RECD   real-ear coupler difference
REIG   real-ear insertion gain
REIR   real-ear insertion response
REOR   real-ear occluded response
REUG   real-ear unaided gain
REUR   real-ear unaided response
RIC   receiver in the canal
RITA   receiver in the aid
RITE   receiver in the ear
Rx   recommendations

SAV   Select-a-Vent
SDS   speech discrimination score
SL   sensation level
SNHL   sensorineural hearing loss
SNR   signal to noise ratio
SPL   sound pressure level
SSD   single side deafness

SSPL   saturation sound pressure level
SRT   speech reception threshold
Sx   symptom

TD   threshold of discomfort
TE   test ear
THD   total harmonic distortion
TM   tympanic membrane
Tx   treatment

UCL   uncomfortable loudness level

VC   volume control

WDRC   wide dynamic range compression
WNL   within normal limits
WR   word recognition

Recommended Reading Material

Audiology: Science to Practice, Third Edition, by Steven Kramer and David K. Brown

Audiology Workbook, Third Edition, by Steven Kramer and Larry H. Small

Basic Audiometry Learning Manual, Second Edition, by Mark DeRuiter and Virginia Ramachandran

Custom Earmold Manual, by Microsonic, Inc.

Distance Learning for Professionals in Hearing Health Sciences, by International Institute for Hearing Instrument Studies

Essentials of Modern Hearing Aids: Selection, Fitting, Verification, by Todd Ricketts, Ruth Bentler, and H. Gustav Mueller

Fitting and Dispensing Hearing Aids, Second Edition, by Brian Taylor and H. Gustav Mueller

Hearing Aids, by Harvey Dillon

Hearing Instrument Science and Fitting Practice, by Robert E. Sandlin

Masking: Practical Applications of Masking Principles and Procedures, by Linda L. Donaldson

Modern Hearing Aids: Pre-fitting and Selection Considerations, by Todd Ricketts, Ruth Bentler, and H. Gustav Mueller

Modern Hearing Aids: Verification, Outcome Measures, and Follow-up, by Todd Ricketts, Ruth Bentler, and H. Gustav Mueller

Pure-Tone Audiometry and Masking, by Maureen Valente

The Audiogram Workbook, by Sharon T. Hepfner

APPENDIX

Module Quiz Answers

MODULE 1 QUIZ ANSWERS

1. B
2. C
3. C
4. D
5. A
6. B
7. A
8. B
9. B
10. D
11. B
12. B
13. B
14. D
15. B
16. A
17. C
18. B
19. B
20. C
21. B
22. A
23. D
24. C
25. D
26. B
27. C
28. E
29. A
30. E

4. B
5. D
6. B
7. C
8. B
9. A
10. D

MODULE 3 QUIZ ANSWERS

1. C
2. B
3. D
4. A
5. D
6. A
7. C
8. A
9. B
10. D
11. A
12. D
13. B
14. D
15. B
16. A
17. A
18. B
19. A
20. D

MODULE 2 QUIZ ANSWERS

1. C
2. B
3. D

MODULE 4 QUIZ ANSWERS

1. B
2. B
3. D

4. A
5. D
6. A
7. C
8. B
9. A

10. D
11. B
12. D
13. B
14. D
15. B

APPENDIX A

State Hearing Aid Dispenser Licensing Department Information

ALABAMA
Hearing Instrument Dealers Board
400 S. Union St., Suite 235-B
Montgomery, AL 36104-4361
http://www.alabamahidb.us/index.html
Phone: (334) 593-3777
Email: HIDB@ATT.NET

ALASKA
Regulation of Hearing Aid Dealers
P.O. Box 110806
Juneau, AK 99811-0806
https://www.commerce.alaska.gov/web
    /cbpl/professionallicensing/hearingaid
    dealers.aspx
Phone: (907) 465-2695
Fax: (907) 465-2974

ARIZONA
Arizona Department of Health Services
Division of Licensing Services—Bureau of
    Special Licensing
150 North 18th #400
Phoenix, AZ 85007
http://www.azdhs.gov/licensing/special
    /index.php#speech-hearing-home
Phone: (602) 364-2079
Fax: (602) 364-4769
Email: Special.Licensing@azdhs.gov

ARKANSAS
Arkansas Board of Hearing Instrument
    Dispensers
PO Box 219
Jacksonville, Arkansas 72078
Phone: (501) 241-1120
Fax: (501) 241-0599

http://www.arkansas.gov/directory/detail2
    .cgi?ID=978

CALIFORNIA
Speech-Language Pathology & Audiology &
    Hearing Aid Dispensers Board
SLPAHADB
2005 Evergreen St., Suite 2100
Sacramento, CA 95815
http://www.speechandhearing.ca.gov
    /contact_us.shtml
Phone: (916) 263-2666
Fax: (916) 263-2668
Email: speechandhearing@dca.ca.gov

COLORADO
Office of Hearing Aid Provider Licensure
1560 Broadway #1350
Denver, CO 80202
https://www.colorado.gov/pacific/dora
    /Hearing_Aid_Provider
Phone: (303) 894-7800
Fax: (303) 894-7764

CONNECTICUT
Connecticut Department of Public Health
HIS Licensure
410 Capitol Ave, MS#12APP
P.O. Box 340308
Hartford, CT 06134-0308
http://www.dph.state.ct.us
Phone: (860) 509-7603

DELAWARE
Delaware Board of SLP/AUD/HAD
861 Silver Lake Blvd, Ste. 203 Cannon
    Building

Dover, DE 19904
https://dpr.delaware.gov/boards/speech
  audio/
Phone: (302) 744-4500
Fax: (302) 739-2711
Email: customerservice.dpr@state.de.us

District of Columbia
Hearing Aid Dealers Licensing
899 North Capitol Street, NE, Washington,
  DC 20002
Phone: (877) 672-2174
Fax: (202) 727-8471
https://dchealth.dc.gov/

FLORIDA
Florida Board of Hearing Aid Specialists
4052 Bald Cypress Way
Bin C-08
Tallahassee, FL 32399-3258
http://www.doh.state.fl.us http://www.doh
  .state.fl.us/mqa/HearingAid/index.html
Phone: (850) 245-4474
Fax: (850) 921-5389

GEORGIA
Georgia Board of Hearing Aid Dealers and
  Dispensers
237 Coliseum Drive
Macon, GA 31217-2440
http://www.sos.georgia.gov/plb/hearingaid
Phone: (478) 207-2440
Fax: (866) 888-7127

HAWAII
Department of Commerce & Consumer Affairs
Attn: HADF
P.O. Box 3469
Honolulu, HI 96801
http://cca.hawaii.gov/pvl/programs
  /hearing/
Phone: (808) 586-2698
Email: hearingaid@dcca.hawaii.gov

IDAHO
Idaho Bureau of Occupational Licenses
  Speech & Hearing Services Licensing
  Board
700 W. State St.

Boise, ID 83720
Mailing Address:
PO Box 83720
Boise, ID 83720-0063
https://ibol.idaho.gov/IBOL/BoardPage
  .aspx?Bureau=SHS
Phone: (208) 334-3233
Fax: (208) 334-3945
Email: ibol@ibol.idaho.gov

ILLINOIS
Illinois Department of Public Health
Hearing Instrument Program
535 W. Jefferson St., Third Floor
Springfield, IL 62761
http://dph.illinois.gov/licensing-certification
  ?page=1
Phone: (217) 524-2396
Fax: (217) 524-4201
Email: dph.visionandhearing@illinois.gov

INDIANA
Indiana Professional Licensing Agency
Attn: Hearing Aid Dealer Committee
402 West Washington Street Room W072
Indianapolis, IN 46204
http://www.in.gov/pla/had.htm
Phone: (317) 234-2067
Email: pla4@pla.in.gov

IOWA
Bureau of Professional Licensure
Iowa Department of Public Health
Lucas State Office Bldg., 5th Floor
321 East 12th Street
Des Moines, IA 50319-0075
http://idph.iowa.gov/Licensure
  /Iowa-Board-of-Hearing-Aid-Dispensers
Phone: (515) 281-0254
Fax: (515) 281-3121

KANSAS
Kansas Board of Hearing Aid Examiners
P.O. Box 232
Garnett, KS 66032
Email: zack.miller@ks.gov
http://www.kbhae.com
Phone: (785) 448-2134
Fax: (785) 448-2166

KENTUCKY

Kentucky Licensing Board for Specialists in
   Hearing Instruments
911 Leawood Dr.
Frankfort, KY 40601
http://his.ky.gov/Pages/default.aspx
Phone: (502) 782-8807
Fax: (502) 696-3853
Email: HIS@ky.gov

LOUISIANA

Louisiana Board of Hearing Aid Dealers
308 Gregory Dr.
Luling, LA 70070
Email: rblbhad@aol.com
https://wwwcfprd.doa.louisiana.gov
   /boardsandcommissions/viewRulesAnd
   Regulations.cfm?board=16
Phone: (405) 420-5424

MAINE

Board of Speech, Audiology, and Hearing
35 State House Station
Augusta, ME 04333-0035
http://www.maine.gov/pfr/professional
   licensing/professions/speech_audiology
   _hearing_aid/ Phone: (207) 624-8626
Fax: (207) 624-8637

MARYLAND

Maryland Department of Health
Board of Audiologists, Hearing Aid Dispens-
   ers & Speech Language Pathologists
Metro Executive Building
4201 Patterson Ave
Baltimore, MD 21215
http://www.mdboardaudhadslp.org/
Phone: (410) 764-4725
Fax: (410) 358-0273

MASSACHUSETTS

Division of Professional Licensing
Board of Registration of Hearing Instrument
   Specialists
1000 Washington Street, Suite 7th Floor
Boston, MA 02118-6100
http://www.mass.gov/ocabr/licensee/dpl
   -boards/he/forms/
Phone: (617) 727-1945

MICHIGAN

Licensing and Regulatory Affairs
Bureau of Professional Licensing
P.O. Box 30670
Lansing, MI 48909
http://www.michigan.gov/lara/0,4601,7
   -154-72600_72602_72731_72868---,00
   .html
Phone: (517) 241-9288

MINNESOTA

Minnesota Department of Health
Health Occupations Program
P.O. Box 64882
St. Paul, MN 55164-0882
http://www.health.state.mn.us
Phone: (651) 201-3731
Fax: (651) 201-3839
Email: health.hop@state.mn.us

MISSISSIPPI

MSDH Professional Licensure Division
P.O. Box 1700
Jackson, MS 39215-1700
http://www.msdh.ms.gov
Phone: (601)364-7360
Fax: (601)364-5057

MISSOURI

Board of Examiners for Hearing Instru-
   ment Specialists
3605 Missouri Blvd
P.O. Box 1335
Jefferson City, MO 65102-1335
http://www.pr.mo.gov/hearing.asp
Phone: (573) 751-0240
Fax: (573) 526-3856
Email: behis@pr.mo.gov

MONTANA

Montana Board of Hearing Aid Dispensers
Montana Department of Labor and Industry
301 S. Park Ave.
Helena, MT 59620
http://www.hearingaid.mt.gov/had
Phone: (406) 841-2395
Fax: (406) 841-2305

NEBRASKA
DHHS, Public Health Licensure Unit
P.O. Box 94986
Lincoln, NE 68509-4986
http://dhhs.ne.gov/publichealth/pages/crl
HISHome.aspx
Phone: (402) 471-2299
Fax: (402) 471-3577
Email: michelle.humlicek@nebraska.gov

NEVADA
State of Nevada Speech-Pathology, Audiol-
ogy, and Hearing Aid Dispensing Board
P.O. Box 34540
Reno, NV 89533-4540
http://www.nvspeechhearing.org/
Phone: (775) 787-3421
Fax: (775) 746-4105

NEW HAMPSHIRE
Board of Hearing Care Providers
121 South Fruit Street
Concord, NH 03301
https://www.oplc.nh.gov/hearing-care/in
dex.htm
Phone: (603) 271-9482
Fax: (603) 271-6702
Email: hearingcare@oplc.nh.gov

NEW JERSEY
Hearing Aid Dispensers Examining
Committee
Renee Clark Executive Director
P.O. Box 45038
Newark, NJ 07101
http://www.njconsumeraffairs.gov/had
/Pages/default.aspx
Phone: (973) 504-6331

NEW MEXICO
Speech-Language Pathology, Audiology and
Hearing Aid Dispensing Practices Board
Toney Anaya Building
2550 Cerrillos Road, Second Floor
Santa Fe, NM 87505
http://www.rld.state.nm.us/boards/Speech
_Language_Pathology_Audiology_and
_Hearing_Aid_Dispensing_Practices.aspx
Phone: (505) 476-4622

Fax: (505) 476-4545
Email: http://speech/Hearing@state.nm.us

NEW YORK
New York State—Department of State
Division of Licensing Services
P.O. Box 22001
Albany, NY 12201-2001
http://www.dos.ny.gov/licensing/hearin
gaid/hearingaid.html
Phone: (518) 474-4429
Fax: (518) 473-6648

NORTH CAROLINA
NC State Hearing Aid Dealers and Fitters
Board
3801 Lake Boone Trail, Ste 190
Raleigh, NC 27607
http://www.nchalb.org/
Phone: (919) 834-3661
Email: info@nchalb.org

NORTH DAKOTA
North Dakota Board of Hearing Aid
Specialists
825 SW 25th Street
Fargo, ND 58103
https://www.governor.nd.gov/boards
/BoardDetails.aspx?boardid=43
Phone: (701) 237-9977

OHIO
Ohio Speech and Hearing Professionals Board
77 South High Street
Columbus, OH 43215
http://shp.ohio.gov/
Phone: (855) 405-5514

OKLAHOMA
Hearing Aid Dealers and Fitters Licensing
Program
Consumer Health Service
PO Box 268815
Oklahoma City, OK 73126
https://www.ok.gov/health/Protective
_Health/Consumer_Health_Service
/Hearing_Aid_Dealers_&_Fitters_Licens
ing_Program/
Phone: (405) 271-5779

Fax: (405) 271-5286
Email: CHSLincensing@health.ok.gov

OREGON

Oregon Health Licensing Office
Advisory Council on Hearing Aids
1430 Tandem Ave NE
Suite 180
Salem, OR 97301
http://www.oregon.gov/oha/PH/HLO
/Pages/Board-Advisory-Council-Hearing
-Aids-License.aspx
Phone: (503) 378-8667
Fax: (503) 373-2024
Email: hlo.info@state.or.us

PENNSYLVANIA

Pennsylvania Department of Health
Hearing Aid Registration Program
132 Kline Plaza, Suite A
Harrisburg, PA 17104
http://www.health.pa.gov/facilities/Laws
%20and%20Regulations/Hearing-Aid
-Regulation-Program-Laws/Pages/Hearing
_Aid_Main.aspx#.WrKFHOjwaUn
Phone: (717) 783-8078
Fax: (717) 772-0232
Email: ra-mmunityprogramlicensure@pa.gov

RHODE ISLAND

Rhode Island Board of Hearing Aid
Dealers & Fitters
Rhode Island Department of Health
3 Capitol Hill
Providence, RI 02908
http://health.ri.gov/licenses/detail.php?id
=226#one
Phone: (401) 222-2828

SOUTH CAROLINA

South Carolina Department of Health and
Environmental Control
2600 Bull Street
Columbia, SC 29201
http://www.scdhec.gov/Health/FHPF
/HealthFacilityRegulationsLicensing
/HealthcareFacilityLicensing/Fa
cilitySpecificInfo/HearingAidSpecialist/
Phone: (803)-545-4370

SOUTH DAKOTA

South Dakota Board of Hearing Aid Dispensers & Audiologists
810 N. Main #298
Spearfish, SD 57783
http://doh.sd.gov/Boards/audiology/Licens
ing.aspx
Phone: (605) 642-1600
Fax: (605) 722-1006
Email: proflic@rushmore.com

TENNESSEE

Department of Health
Council for Hearing Instruments Specialists
665 Mainstream Drive
2nd Floor
Nashville, TN 37243
https://www.tn.gov/health/health-program
-areas/health-professional-boards/his
-board/his-board/about.html
Phone: (615) 741-5735

TEXAS

Texas Department of Licensing and
Regulation
P.O. Box 12157
Austin, TX 78711
https://www.tdlr.texas.gov/hearing/hearing
.htm
Phone: (512) 463-6599
Email: CS.Hearing.Fitters@tdlr.texas.gov

UTAH

Utah Division of Occupational and Profes-
sional Licensing
Hearing Instrument
160 East 300 South
Salt Lake City, UT 84114
http://dopl.utah.gov/licensing/hearing
_instrument.html
Phone: (801) 530-6628
Fax: (801) 530-6511
Email: doplweb@utah.gov

VERMONT

Office of Professional Regulation—Hearing
Aid Dispensers
Colin Benjamin
Director

89 Main Street, 3rd Floor
Montpelier VT 05620-3402
https://www.sec.state.vt.us/professional
-regulation/list-of-professions/hearing
-aid-dispensers.aspx
Phone: (802) 828-5434

VIRGINIA

Virginia Department of Professional &
Occupational Regulation
9960 Maryland Drive, Suite 400
Richmond, VA 23233-1485
http://www.dpor.virginia.gov/Boards/HAS
-Opticians/
Phone: (804) 367-8509
Fax: (804) 245-9693
Email: BCHOPLicensing@dpor.virginia.gov

WASHINGTON

Hearing and Speech Credentialing
P.O. Box 47877
Olympia, WA 98504-7877
https://www.doh.wa.gov/LicensesPer
mitsandCertificates/ProfessionsNewRe
neworUpdate/HearingAidSpecialist
/ApplicationsandForms
Phone: (360) 236-4700

WEST VIRGINIA

Board of Hearing Aid Dealers and Fitters
703 Peoples Building
179 Summers Street

Charleston, WV 25301
http://www.wvdhhr.org/wvbhadf/
Phone: (304) 558-3527
Email: boardofhearingaiddealers@frontier
.com

WISCONSIN

Wisconsin Hearing and Speech Examining
Board
1400 E. Washington Ave.
P.O. Box 8935
Madison, WI 53703
https://dsps.wi.gov/Pages/RulesStatutes
/HAS.aspx
Phone: (608) 266-2112

WYOMING

Wyoming Board of Hearing Aid Specialists
Debra Bridges
2001 Capitol Ave
Room 104
Cheyenne, WY 82002
http://hearingaid.wyo.gov/
Phone: (307) 777-3628
Fax: (307) 777-3508
Email: amanda.best@wyo.gov

APPENDIX B

Spondee Word List

- GREYHOUND
- AIRPLANE
- SCHOOLBOY
- INKWELL
- OATMEAL
- WHITEWASH
- TOOTHBRUSH
- PANCAKE
- FAREWELL
- MOUSETRAP
- GRANDSON
- EARDRUM
- DRAWBRIDGE
- HEADLIGHT
- DOORMAT
- BIRTHDAY
- HOTHOUSE
- DUCKPOND
- DAYBREAK
- SIDEWALK
- SUNSET
- HOTDOG
- PLAYGROUND
- PADLOCK
- GRANDSON

- MUSHROOM
- DAYBREAK
- HARDWARE
- DOORMAT
- WORKSHOP
- WOODWORK
- HORSESHOE
- ARMCHAIR
- STAIRWAY
- BASEBALL
- COWBOY
- STAIRWAY
- OATMEAL
- COWBOY
- RAILROAD
- ICEBERG
- BASEBALL
- NORTHWEST
- PADLOCK
- RAILROAD
- HARDWARE
- PLAYGROUND
- WHITEWASH
- STAIRWAY
- ARMCHAIR

PHONETICALLY BALANCED WORD LISTS—NU 6

List 1	List 2
Laud	Pick
Boat	Room
Pool	Nice
Nag	Said
Limb	Fail
Shout	South
Sub	White
Vine	Keep
Dime	Dead
Goose	Loaf
Whip	Dab
Tough	Numb
Puff	Juice
Keen	Chief
Death	Merge
Sell	Wag
Take	Rain
Fall	Witch
Raise	Soap
Third	Young
Gap	Ton
Fat	Keg
Met	Calm
Jar	Tool
Door	Pike
Love	Mill
Sure	Hush
Knock	Shack
Choice	Read
Hash	Rot
Lot	Hate
Raid	Live
Hurl	Book
Moon	Voice
Page	Gaze
Yes	Pad
Reach	Thought
King	Bought
Home	Turn
Rag	Chair
Which	Lore
Week	Bite
Size	Haze
Mode	Match
Bean	Learn

PHONETICALLY BALANCED WORD LISTS—NU 6 *(continued)*

List 1	List 2
■ Tip	■ Shawl
■ Chalk	■ Deep
■ Jail	■ Gin
■ Burn	■ Goal
■ Kite	■ Far

APPENDIX C

Blank Audiograms

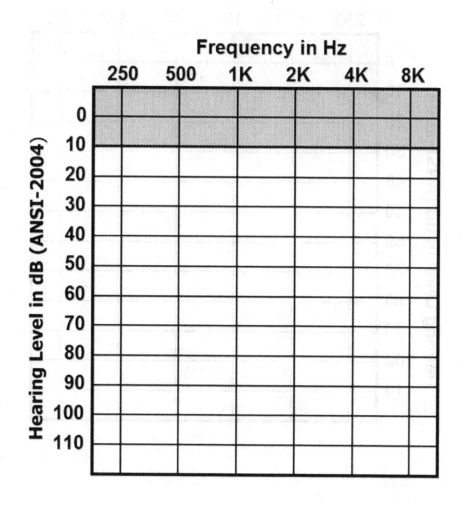

Frequency in Hz

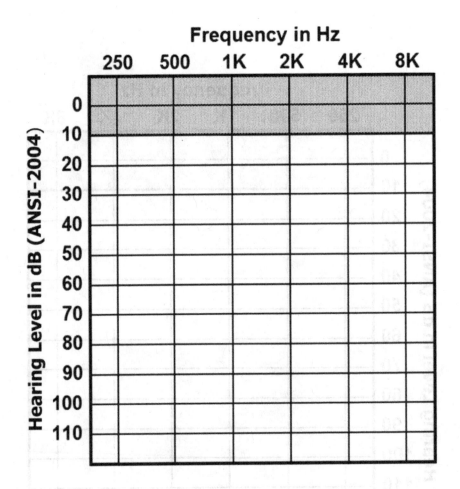

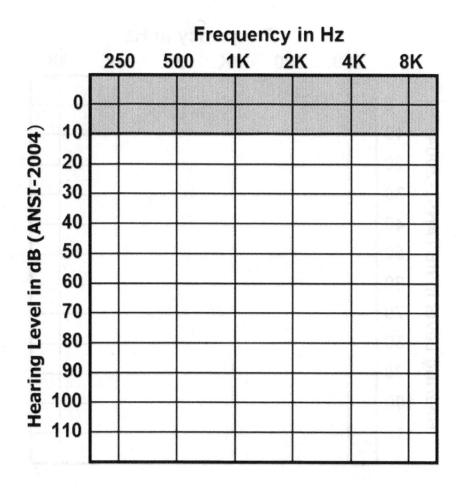

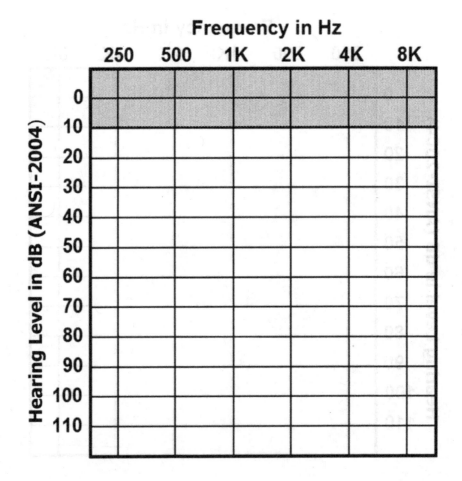

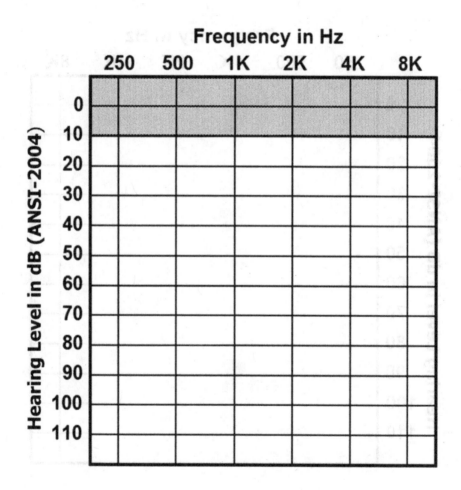

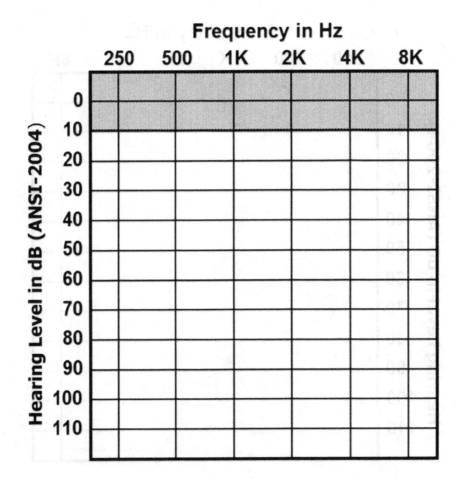

APPENDIX D

Hearing Aid Delivery Checklist

1. *Otoscopic Inspection:* _____

2. *Verification*

___ In situ audiometry (choose 1)   ___ Subjective assessment

___ Speech mapping (choose 1)   ___ Check for proper fit

___ Real-ear measurement (choose 1)

3. *Hearing Instrument Use*

___ Identification of the right/left   ___ Telephone use

___ Insertion and removal of battery   ___ User controls VC/MMB/remote, etc.

___ Insertion/removal of hearing aids/ earmolds   ___ Counseling on comfort

4. *Hearing Aid Maintenance and Care*

___ Battery type, size, and life   ___ Dri-Aid kit/dry and store

___ Battery door open when not in use   ___ Troubleshooting

___ Battery compartment when not in use   ___ Proper cleaning: brush, pick, etc.

___ Battery storage and disposal   ___ Proper storage of aids

___ Where/how to purchase batteries   ___ Keep away from pets and small children

___ Battery ingestion dangers, hotline #

___ Advise not to expose aids to hairspray, water, oil, dust, etc.   ___ Troubleshooting, owner's manual

5. *Counseling on Expectations and Limitations*

___ Realistic expectations   ___ Motivation to use hearing aids

___ Family support   ___ Learning to listen again

___ Methods of adjustment to amplification

___ Aural rehabilitation

___ Wearing schedule

___ Discuss COSI

6. *Service*

___ Expiration of warranty

___ Explanation of coverage

___ Schedule follow-up appointments

___ Review and complete the purchase agreement, provide copy to patient

APPENDIX E

Troubleshooting a Hearing Aid

1. **Wash hands** before handling the Hearing Aid and handle with a tissue or sanitary cloth
2. Wash hands and perform an **Otoscopic Evaluation** on the patient if he/she is present
3. Wash hands and perform a **Visual Inspection** of the Hearing Aid
4. Check and test the **Battery**
5. Use your otoscope or magnifying glass and perform a more **in-depth inspection** of the hearing aid. Check Microphone, Receiver, Battery Contact, VC, Memory Button, Switches, etc.
6. Using your Stethoscope, perform a **listening check** of the device verifying that any and all buttons/switches/VC are functioning properly. Open and close battery door as well and listen for static, intermittency, etc.
7. Once you have identified the problem, explain how you would correct it.
8. Perform **a 2-cc coupler measurement** of the device in a Hearing Aid Test box to verify that the instrument is up to manufacturer specifications compared with the spec sheet provided by the manufacturer.
9. Sanitize the HA and fit the device on the patient.

APPENDIX F

FDA Red Flags Cheat Sheet

1. D: Drainage (past 90 days)
2. D: Dizziness
3. D: Deformity of the ear
4. C: Conductive hearing loss
5. C: Cerumen or foreign body in the ear canal
6. U: Unilateral hearing loss (past 90 days)
7. P: Pain or discomfort
8. S: Sudden or rapid hearing loss (past 90 days)

Appendix F

FDA Red Flags Cheat Sheet

Index